Pocket Prescriber

Timothy R.J. Nicholson
MBBS (London), BSc (London), MSc (Oxon), MRCP (UK)
Having trained in General Medicine
at the Hammersmith Hospital, London,
he is currently training in Psychiatry
at the Maudsley Hospital, London

Editorial Advisor:
Donald R.J. Singer BMedBiol, MD, FRCP
Professor of Clinical Pharmacology, Clinical
Pharmacology Section, Leicester–Warwick
Medical Schools, University of Warwick,
Coventry, UK

Hodder Arnold

A MEMBER OF THE HODDER HEADLINE GROUP

First published in Great Britain in 2004 by
Arnold, a member of the Hodder Headline Group,
338 Euston Road, London NW1 3BH

http://www.hoddereducation.co.uk

Distributed in the United States of America by
Oxford University Press Inc.,
198 Madison Avenue, New York, NY10016
Oxford is a registered trademark of Oxford University Press

British Library Cataloguing in Publication Data
A catalogue record for this book is available from the British Library

Library of Congress Cataloging-in-Publication Data
A catalog record for this book is available from the Library of Congress

ISBN-10: 0 340 81151 X

ISBN-13: 978 0 340 81151 1

4 5 6 7 8 9 10

Commissioning Editor: Georgina Bentliff
Development Editor: Heather Smith
Project Editor: Anke Ueberberg
Production Controller: Lindsay Smith
Cover Design: Amina Dudhia

Typeset in 8/10 pt Sabon by Charon Tec Pvt. Ltd, Chennai, India
Printed and bound in Spain

What do you think about this book? Or any other Arnold title?
Please send your comments to **www.hoddereducation.co.uk**

CONTENTS

Acknowledgements   v
Foreword   vii
How to use this book   ix

Common/useful drugs   1

Drug selection   127
Antibiotics   128
Hypertension management   137
Asthma   139
Analgesia   140
Palliative care and subcutaneous pumps   142
Antiemetics   145
Alcohol withdrawal   147

How to prescribe   149
Insulin   150
Anticoagulants   154
Thrombolysis   161
Controlled drugs   163

Miscellaneous   165
Intravenous fluids   166
Steroids   169
Sedation/Sleeping tablets   171
Benzodiazepines   173
Side-effect profiles   174
Cytochrome P450   176

Medical emergencies   177
Acute MI (AMI) and acute coronary syndrome (ACS)   178
Acute LVF   181
Accelerated hypertension   181
Anaphylaxis   182

Acute asthma   182
COPD exacerbation   183
Pulmonary embolism   184
Epilepsy   185
DKA   186
HONK   187
↓Glucose   188
Thyrotoxic crisis   188
Myxoedema coma   189
Addisonian crisis   190
Electrolyte disturbances   190
Overdoses   192
Coma   197
Common laboratory reference values   197

Index   201

Algorithms

Bradycardia algorithm   *Outside front cover flap*
Narrow complex tachycardia algorithm   *Inside front cover flap*
Broad complex tachycardia algorithm   *Inside front cover*
Atrial fibrillation algorithm   *Inside back cover*
ALS universal algorithm   *Outside back cover flap*

ACKNOWLEDGEMENTS

This book is dedicated to my family and friends as well as all the inspirational teachers I have been lucky enough to learn from over the years, in particular John Youle, Katie Blackman, Jerry Kirk, Carol Black, Huw Beynon, Martin Rossor, Michael Trimble and Maria Ron. Particular thanks for their help and time to Anand and Subbu, Houman Ashrafian, Nick Bateman, Roger Cross, Jonny Crowston, Chris Denton, Emma Derritt-Smith, Paul Dilworth, Nick Eynon-Lewis, Fahad Farooqi, Catherine Farrow, Roger Fernandes, Arosha Fernando, Denise Forth, Jack Galliford, Hamid Ghodse, Natasha Gilani, Peter Hargreaves, Rick Holliman, Sudhesh Kumar, Graham MacGregor, Mel Mahadevan, Omar Malik, Narbeh Melikan, Alli Morton, Neil Muchatuta, Dev Mukerjee, Gideon Paul, Tejal Patel, Rahul Patel, Rakita Patel, Annabel Price, Amar Sharif, Bran Sivakumar, Sian Stanley, Richard Stratton, Henry Squire, Mike Travis and Aaron Vallance.

Special thanks to Helen Galley.

The information in this book has been collated from many sources, including manufacturer's information sheets ('SPCs' – summary of product characteristics sheets), the British National Formulary (BNF), national and international guidelines, as well as numerous pharmacology and general medical books, journals and papers. Where information is not consistent between these sources that from the SPCs has been taken as definitive.

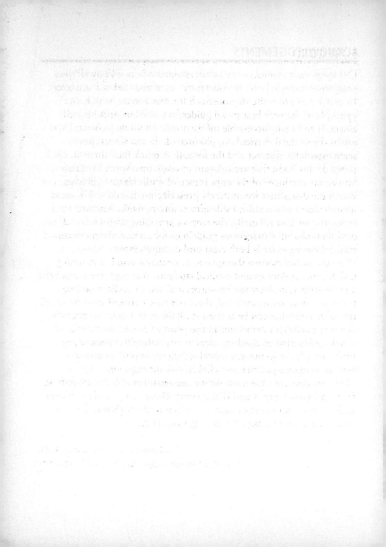

FOREWORD

Contemporary medical practice necessitates a broad knowledge
drug treatments, which are constantly being updated and modifie
I am delighted to write the foreword for this volume which, in the
principle of the very best travel guides, is small but packed with
essential and easily accessible information. Of all the subjects that
are in the medical curriculum, pharmacology can sometimes
seem especially abstract and theoretical. A quick flick through the
pages of this book that are relevant to one's own speciality is an
immediate reminder of the importance of understanding the ways in
which the drugs that we routinely prescribe are handled. The clear
identification of hazardous side-effects and potential interactions is
especially welcome. Finally, the section providing current
information and management guidelines for commonly encountered
medical emergencies is both clear and comprehensive.

  Safe use of the modern therapeutic armamentarium is a daunting
task for junior doctors and medical students. Although there has been
a large growth in electronic resources and some excellent on-line
textbooks have been produced, there remains a critical need for small
reference texts that can be carried at all times and used to check drug
doses or potential interactions at the point of prescription. The
simple precaution of checking facts in any unfamiliar prescribing
situation is likely to prevent mistakes, and exemplifies current
emphasis on safe-practice and clinical risk management.

  I believe that even the most senior specialist could learn something
from this book's pages and that a comprehensive up-to-date volume
such as this is an essential part of any junior doctor's tool kit, and
will prove useful far beyond its target audience.

Professor Carol M. Black CBE
President of the Royal College of Physicians

HOW TO USE THIS BOOK

The aim of this pocket book is to provide the reference information needed for the majority of prescriptions made by a junior doctor, along with practical prescribing advice. By its nature, it will omit much detail, which can of course be found in other sources. The information is highly keyed and condensed, but once you are familiar with the format, it should be quick to use, save you much time, and enable more frequent checks and subsequently safer prescribing.

IMPORTANT INFORMATION

This book is not comprehensive. Not all features of each drug (in particular, side effects and interactions) are mentioned. Only important and need to-know information is included.

If you need further information about specific drugs, please consult other sources, such as manufacturers' information sheets, the *British National Formulary* (BNF), your pharmacy, and your clinical colleagues.

It must also be noted that this book is based on current prescribing practice in the UK on drug nomenclature, formulations, doses and guidelines for use within this. Readers in countries outside the UK should ensure that information in the book is used in the context of their national advice on medical practice and prescribing.

Any errors noted and comments on how to improve this book will be received gratefully. Please write with your comments or suggestions to Dr Timothy K.J. Nicholson, Pocket Prescriber, c/o Hodder Arnold, Health Sciences, 338 Euston Road, London NW1 3BH, UK or email pocketprescriber@hodder.co.uk.

STANDARD LAYOUT OF DRUGS

DRUG/TRADE NAME

Class/action: More information is given for generic forms, especially for the original and most commonly used drug(s) of each class.

Use: use^x.

CI: contraindications; **L** (liver failure), **R** (renal failure), **H** (heart failure), **P** (pregnancy), **B** (breastfeeding). *Hypersensitivity to the drug is assumed too obvious to mention.*

Caution: **L** (liver failure), **R** (renal failure), **H** (heart failure), **P** (pregnancy), **B** (breastfeeding), **E** (elderly patients).

SE: side effects; listed in order of frequency encountered. Common/important side effects set in **bold**.

Warn: information to give to patients before starting drug.

Monitor: parameters that need to be monitored during treatment.

Interactions: included only if very common or potentially serious; ↑/↓**P450** (induces/inhibits cytochrome P450 metabolism), **W+** (increases effect of warfarin), **W−** (decreases effect of warfarin).

Dose: dose^x (for Use^x as above).

Important points highlighted at end of drug entry.

Use/dose^{NICE}: National Institute of Clinical Excellence guidelines exist for the drug (details often in BNF, or see www.nice.org.uk).

Dose^{BNF}: regime for dosing is complicated; please refer to BNF or product literature/manufacturer's information sheets.

* links between information within an individual drug entry are done using asterisks.

Sections are included only if relevant to the drug in question. Trade names are given only if found regularly on drug charts or if non-proprietary (generic, non-trade-name) drug does not exist yet. *Doses given are for adults only.*

KEY

☠ Potential dangers highlighted with skull and cross-bones

▼ New drug or new indication under intense surveillance by Committee on Safety of Medicines (CSM): *important to report all suspected drug reactions via Yellow Card scheme* (accurate as going to press: from January 2004 CSM list)

☺ *Good for:* reasons to give a certain drug when choice exists
☹ *Bad for:* reasons to not give a certain drug when choice exists
⇒ Causes/goes to
∴ Therefore
Δ Change/disturbance
Ψ Psychiatric
↑ Increase/high
↓ Decrease/low

> ↑/↓ electrolytes refers to serum levels, unless stated otherwise.

DOSES

od	once daily
bd	twice daily
tds	three times daily
qds	four times daily
nocte	at night
mane	in the morning
prn	as required
stat	at once

ROUTES

im	intramuscular
inh	inhaled
iv	intravenous
ivi	intravenous infusion
neb	via nebuliser
po	oral
pr	rectal
sc	subcutaneous
top	topical

> Routes are presumed po, unless stated otherwise.

ABBREVIATIONS

AAC	antibiotic-associated colitis
Ab	antibody
ACE-i	ACE inhibitor
ACh	acetylcholine
ACS	acute coronary syndrome
AF	atrial fibrillation
Ag	antigen
ALL	acute lymphoblastic leukaemia
AMI	acute myocardial infarction
AMTS	abbreviated mental test score (same as MTS)
5-ASA	5-aminosalicylic acid
AV	arteriovenous
AVM	arteriovenous malformation
AVN	atrioventricular node
ARDS	adult respiratory distress syndrome
ARF	acute renal failure
AS	aortic stenosis
ASAP	as soon as possible
BBB	bundle branch block
BCT	broad complex tachycardia
BF	blood flow
BG	serum blood glucose; *see also CBG*
BHS	British Hypertension Society
BIH	benign intracranial hypertension
BM	bone marrow (NB: BM is often used, confusingly, to signify finger-prick glucose; CBG (capillary blood glucose) is used for this purpose in this book)
BMI	body mass index = weight (kg)/height (m)^2
BP	blood pressure
BPH	benign prostatic hypertrophy
BTS	British Thoracic Society
Bx	biopsy
C	constipation
Ca	cancer (NB: calcium is abbreviated to Ca^{++})
CAH	congenital adrenal hyperplasia
CBF	cerebral blood flow
CBG	capillary blood glucose (finger-prick testing) (NB: BM is often used to denote this, but this is confusing and less accurate and thus not used in this book)

CCF	congestive cardiac failure
cf	compared with
CI	contraindicated
CK	creatine kinase
CLL	chronic lymphocytic leukaemia
CML	chronic myelogenous leukaemia
CMV	cytomegalovirus
CNS	central nervous system
CO	cardiac output
COPD	chronic obstructive pulmonary disease
COX	cyclo-oxygenase
CPR	cardiopulmonary resuscitation
CRF	chronic renal failure
CSF	cerebrospinal fluid
CSM	Committee on Safety of Medicines
CVA	cerebrovascular accident
CVP	central venous pressure
CXR	chest X-ray
D	diarrhoea
$D_{1/2/3\,...}$	dopamine receptor subtype 1/2/3 ...
DA	dopamine
DCT	distal convoluted tubule
dfx	defects
DI	diabetes insipidus
DIGAMI	glucose, insulin and potassium intravenous infusion used in acute myocardial infarction
DKA	diabetic ketoacidosis
DM	diabetes mellitus
DMARD	disease-modifying anti-rheumatoid arthritis drug
dt	due to
D&V	diarrhoea and vomiting
Dx	diagnosis
EBV	Epstein–Barr virus
ECG	electrocardiogram
ECT	electroconvulsive therapy
ENT	ear, nose and throat
EØ	eosinophils
ESC	European Society of Cardiology
ESR	erythrocyte sedimentation rate
exac	exacerbates
FBC	full blood count

FFP	fresh frozen plasma
FiO_2	inspired O_2 concentration
FMF	Familial Mediterranean Fever
fx	effects
GABA	gamma aminobutyric acid
GBS	Guillain–Barré syndrome
GCS	Glasgow coma scale
GI	gastrointestinal
GIK	glucose, insulin and K^+ infusion
G6PD	glucose-6-phosphate dehydrogenase
GU	genitourinary
HB	heart block
Hct	haematocrit
HDL	high-density lipoprotein
HF	heart failure
HIV	human immunodeficiency virus
HMG-CoA	3-hydroxy-3-methyl-glutaryl coenzyme A
H(O)CM	hypertrophic (obstructive) cardiomyopathy
HONK	hyperosmolar non-ketotic state
HSV	herpes simplex virus
5-HT	5-hydroxytryptamine (= serotonin)
HTN	hypertension
HUS	haemolytic uraemic syndrome
Hx	history
IBD	inflammatory bowel disease
IBS	irritable bowel syndrome
ICP	intracranial pressure
ICU	intensive care unit
IHD	ischaemic heart disease
inc	including
IOP	intraocular pressure
ITP	immune/idiopathic thrombocytopoenic purpura
ITU	intensive therapy unit
Ix	investigation
IVDU	intravenous drug user
K^+	potassium (serum levels unless stated otherwise)
LA	long-acting
LBBB	left bundle branch block
LDL	low–density lipoprotein
LF	liver failure
LFTs	liver function tests

LØ	lymphocytes
LP	lumbar puncture
LVF	left ventricular failure
MAOI	monoamine oxidase inhibitor
MAP	mean arterial pressure
MG	myasthenia gravis
MI	myocardial infarction
MMSE	mini mental state examination (scored out of 30)
MØ	macrophages
MR	modified-release (drug preparation)
MRSA	methicillin-resistant *Staphylococcus aureus*
MS	multiple sclerosis
MTS	(abbreviated) mental test score (scored out of 10)
Mx	management
N	nausea
Na$^+$	sodium (serum levels unless stated otherwise)
NA	noradrenaline (norepinephrine)
NBM	nil by mouth
NCT	narrow complex tachycardia
NGT	nasogastric tube
NIV	non-invasive ventilation
NMJ	neuromuscular junction
NØ	neutrophils
NSAID	nonsteroidal anti-inflammatory drug
NSTEMI	non-ST elevation myocardial infarction
N&V	nausea and vomiting
OCD	obsessive compulsive disorder
OD	overdose (*NB: od = once daily*)
PAN	polyarteritis nodosa
PBC	primary biliary cirrhosis
PCOS	polycystic ovary syndrome
PCI	percutaneous coronary intervention (now preferred term for percutaneous transluminal coronary angioplasty (PTCA), which is a subtype of PCI)
PCP	*Pneumocystis carinii* pneumonia
PDA	patent ductus arteriosus
PE	pulmonary embolism
PEG	percutaneous endoscopic gastrostomy
PG(*x*)	prostaglandin (receptor subtype *x*)
phaeo	phaeochromocytoma
PHx	past history (of)

PID	pelvic inflammatory disease
PMR	polymyalgia rheumatica
PO_4	phosphate (serum levels, unless stated otherwise)
PPI	proton pump inhibitor
prn	as required
Pt	platelet(s)
PT	prothrombin time
PTH	parathyroid hormone
PU	peptic ulcer
PUO	pyrexia of unknown origin
PVD	peripheral vascular disease
Px	prophylaxis
QT(c)	QT interval (corrected for rate)
RA	rheumatoid arthritis
RAS	renal artery stenosis
RBF	renal blood flow
RF	renal failure
RR	respiratory rate
RVF	right ventricular failure
Rx	treatment
SAH	subarachnoid haemorrhage
SAN	sinoatrial node
SE(s)	side effect(s)
SIADH	syndrome of inappropriate antidiuretic hormone
SJS	Stevens–Johnson syndrome
SLE	systemic lupus erythematosus
SOA	swelling of ankles
SOB (OE)	shortness of breath (on exertion)
SR	slow–/sustained-release (drug preparation)
SSRI	selective serotonin reuptake inhibitor
SSS	sick sinus syndrome
SVT	supraventricular tachycardia
supp	suppository
T_4	thyroxine ($\uparrow/\downarrow T_4$ = hyper/hypothyroid)
$t_{1/2}$	half-life
TCA	tricyclic antidepressant
TE	thromboembolism
TEDS	thromboembolism deterrent stockings
TEN	toxic epidermal necrolysis
TFTs	thyroid function tests
TG	triglyceride

TNF	tumour necrosis factor
TPMT	thiopurine methyltransferase
TPR	total peripheral resistance
TTP	thrombotic thrombocytopoenic purpura
UC	ulcerative colitis
U&Es	urea and electrolytes
URTI	upper respiratory tract infection
UTI	urinary tract infection
UV	ultraviolet
V	vomiting
VLDL	very low–density lipoprotein
VT	ventricular tachycardia
VZV	varicella zoster virus (chickenpox/shingles)
w	with
WCC	white cell count
w/in	within
wk	week
w/o	without
WPW	Wolf–Parkinson–White syndrome
Wt	weight
xs	excess
ZE	Zollinger–Ellison syndrome

Common/useful drugs

ABCIXIMAB/REOPRO

Antiplatelet agent, monoclonal Ab against Pt glycoprotein IIb/IIIa receptor (involved in Pt aggregation).

Use: IHD as adjunct to aspirin/heparin, esp if high risk ACS and awaiting PCI[NICE].

CI: major (or any intra-cranial/-spinal) surgery/trauma or active internal bleeding w/in 2 months. Also bleeding disorders (esp ↓Pt), CVA w/in 2 years, intracranial disease (neoplasm, aneurysm or AVM), vasculitis, severe HTN, retinopathy (secondary to HTN or DM) **L/R** (if either severe), **B**.

Caution: drugs that ↑bleeding risk, **P**.

SE: bleeding/↓Pt*, N&V, ↓BP, ↓HR, pain (chest, back or pleuritic), fever. Rarely, hypersensitivity, tamponade, respiratory reactions (inc ARDS).

Monitor: FBC*, clotting.

Dose: 250 µg/kg iv over 1 min, then 0.125 µg/kg/min (max 10 µg/min) ivi. Needs concurrent heparin (LMWH is simplest; patients with ACS are usually already on this).

Specialist use only: get senior advice or contact on-call cardiology.

ACAMPROSATE/CAMPRAL EC

Modifies GABA transmission ⇒ ↓pleasurable fx of alcohol ∴ ↓s craving and relapse rate.

Use: maintaining alcohol abstinence.

CI: L (only if severe), **R/P/B**.

SE: GI upset, rash, Δ libido.

Dose: 666 mg tds po if age 18–65 years (avoid outside this age range) and >60 kg (if <60 kg give 666 mg mane then 333 mg noon and nocte). *Start ASAP after alcohol stopped.*

ACETYLCYSTEINE/PARVOLEX

Precursor of glutathione, which detoxifies metabolites of paracetamol.

Use: paracetamol OD.

Caution: asthma*.

SE: allergy: rash, bronchospasm*, anaphylaxis.
Dose: initially 150 mg/kg in 200 ml 5% glucose ivi over
15 min, then 50 mg/kg in 500 ml over 4 h, then 100 mg/kg in 1 l
over 16 h.

See pp. 193–5 for Mx of paracetamol OD and treatment line graph.

ACICLOVIR (previously ACYCLOVIR)

Antiviral. Inhibits DNA polymerase *only in infected cells*: needs
activation by viral thymidine kinase (produced by herpes spp).
Use: *iv*: severe HSV or VZV infections, e.g. meningitis, encephalitis,
in immunocompromised patients (esp HIV – also used for Px);
po/top: mucous membrane, genital, eye infections.
Caution: dehydration*, R/P/B.
SE: at ↑doses: **ARF, encephalopathy** (esp if dehydrated*). Also
hypersensitivity, GI upset, blood disorders, skin reactions,
headache, many nonspecific neurological symptoms. Rarely Ψ
reactions and hepatotoxicity.
Interactions: if systemic Rx, fx ↑d by probenecid, MMF.
Dose: 5 mg/kg tds ivi over 1 h (10 mg/kg if HSV encephalitis or
VZV in immunocompromised patients); po/top^{BNF}.

ivi leaks ⇒ severe local inflammation/ulceration.

ACTIVATED CHARCOAL see Charcoal

ACTRAPID Short-acting soluble insulin; see p. 150 for use.

ADENOSINE

Purine nucleoside. Slows AVN conduction, dilates coronary arteries;
acts on its own specific receptors.
Use: SVT Rx and tachycardia Dx (↓s rate to reveal underlying
rhythm).
CI: **asthma*** (consider verapamil instead). 2nd-/3rd-degree
HB, SSS.
Caution: heart transplant (↓dose), AF/flutter (↑s accessory pathway
conduction).

SE: bronchospasm*, ↓BP, rarely ⇒ ↓↓HR (all usually
transient).

Warn: ⇒ transient flushing, dyspnoea, nausea, angina.

Interactions: fx ↑by **dipyridamole**: ↓initial adenosine dose to
0.5–1 mg and watch for ↑bleeding (*anti-Pt fx of dipyridamole also
↑d by adenosine*). fx ↓d by **theophyllines**.

Dose: 3–6 mg iv stat; double dose and repeat every 1–2 min
until response or significant AV block (max 12 mg/dose). Give via
central or large peripheral vein and attach cardiac monitor.

$t_{1/2}$ <10 s: often needs readministration (esp if given for Rx cf Dx).

ADRENALINE (im/iv)

Sympathomimetic: powerful stimulation of α (vasoconstriction),
β_1 (↑HR, ↑contractility) and β_2 (vasodilation, bronchodilation,
uterine relaxation).

Use: CPR (see ALS universal algorithm in inside back cover),
anaphylaxis. Rarely other causes of bronchospasm or shock (e.g. 2° to
spinal/ epidural anaesthesia).

Caution: cerebrovascular* and heart disease (esp arrhythmias
and HTN), DM, ↑T_4, glaucoma (angle closure), labour (esp 2nd
stage). **E**.

SE: ↑HR, ↑BP, anxiety, sweats, tremor, headache, peripheral
vasoconstriction, arrhythmias, pulmonary oedema (at ↑doses),
N&V, weakness, dizziness, Ψ disturbance, hyperglycaemia,
urinary retention (esp if ↑prostate). Rarely CVA* (2° to HTN:
monitor BP).

Dose: CPR: 1 mg **iv** = 10 ml of 1:**10 000** (100 μg/ml) then flush
with ⩾20 ml saline. *If no iv access, give 2–3 mg via endotracheal
tube.* **Anaphylaxis:** 0.5 mg **im** = 0.5 ml of 1 in **1000** (1 mg/ml);
repeat after 5 min if no response. (If cardiac arrest seems imminent
or concerns over im absorption, give 0.5 mg **iv** *slowly* = 5 ml of
1:**10 000** (100 μg/ml) at 1 ml/min until response – get senior help
first if possible as iv route ⇒ ↑risk of arrhythmias.)

☠Do not confuse 1:1000 (im) with 1:10 000 (iv) solutions.☠

ADVIL see Ibuprofen

AGGRASTAT see Tirofiban; IIb/IIIa inhibitor (anti-Pt drug) for IHD.

ALENDRONATE/FOSAMAX
Bisphosphonate: ↓s bone turnover.
Use: osteoporosis Rx and Px (esp if on corticosteroids).
CI: delayed GI emptying (esp achalasia and oesophageal stricture/other abnormalities), ↓Ca^{++}, **P/B**.
Caution: upper GI disorders (inc gastritis/PU) **R**.
SE: oesophageal reactions*, GI upset/distension, ↓Ca^{++}, ↓PO$_4^-$ (transient), PU, hypersensitivity (esp skin reactions).
Warn: take with full glass of water on an empty stomach ⩾30 min before, and stay upright until, breakfast*.
Dose: 5–10 mg mane^{BNF} (if 10 mg od, can give as once-weekly 70-mg tablet▼).

ALFACALCIDOL
1-α-hydroxycholecalciferol: partially activated vitamin D (1α hydroxy group normally added by kidney), but still requires hepatic (25)-hydroxylation for full activation.
Use: severe vitamin D deficiency, esp 2° to CRF.
CI/SE: ↑Ca^{++}: monitor levels, watch for symptoms (esp N&V).
Dose: 0.25–1 μg od po.

ALLOPURINOL
Xanthine oxidase inhibitor: ↓s uric acid synthesis.
Use: gout Px, esp if urate stones/renal impairment.
CI: acute gout: can worsen – do not start drug during attack (but do not stop drug if acute attack occurs during Rx).
Caution: **R** (↓dose), **L** (monitor LFTs), **P/B**.
SE: GI upset, ☠severe skin reactions☠ (*stop drug if rash develops and allopurinol is implicated* – can reintroduce cautiously if mild reaction and no recurrence). Rarely, neuropathy (and many nonspecific neurological symptoms), blood disorders, RF, hepatotoxicity.
Warn: report rashes, maintain good hydration.
Interactions: ↑s fx of azathioprine and theophyllines. **W+**.

Dose: initially 100 mg od po ($\uparrow$ to max of 900 mg/day in divided doses of up to 300 mg) after food.

Initial Rx can $\uparrow$gout: give colchicine or NSAID (e.g. indometacin or diclofenac – *not aspirin*) as Px until $\geqslant$1 month after urate normalised.

ALPHAGAN see Brimonidine eye drops

ALTEPLASE ((**R**ecombinant) **T**issue-type **P**lasminogen **A**ctivator, rt-PA, TPA)
Recombinant fibrinolytic.
Use: acute **MI**, massive **PE**, acute ischaemic CVA w/in 3 h of onset (specialist use only).
CI/Caution/SE: See pp. 161–3 for use in MI (for other indications see product literature).
Dose: MI: total dose of 100 mg – regimen depends on time since onset of pain: *0–6 h*: 15 mg iv stat, then 50 mg ivi over 30 min, then 35 mg ivi over 60 min; *6–12 h*: 10 mg iv stat, then 50 mg ivi over 60 min, then four further 10 mg ivis, each over 30 min. **PE**: 10 mg iv over 1–2 min then 90 mg ivi over 2 h.

☠$\downarrow$doses if patient <65 kg; see product literature.☠
If MI concurrent unfractionated iv heparin needed for $\geqslant$24 h; see p. 163. Also needed for **PE**; see product literature.

ALUMINIUM HYDROXIDE
Antacid, PO_4-binding agent ($\downarrow$s GI absorption).
Use: dyspepsia, $\uparrow PO_4$ (which can $\uparrow$risk of bone disease; esp good if secondary to RF, when $\uparrow Ca^{++}$ can occur dt $\uparrow$PTH, as other PO_4 binders often contain Ca^{++}).
CI: $\downarrow PO_4$, porphyria.
SE: constipation*. Aluminium can accumulate in RF (esp if dialysis) $\Rightarrow$ $\uparrow$risk of encephalopathy, dementia, osteomalacia.
Dose: 1–2 (500 mg) tablets or 5–10 ml of 4% suspension prn (qds often sufficient). $\uparrow$doses to individual requirements, esp if for $\uparrow PO_4$. Also available as 475 mg capsules as Alucaps (contains $\downarrow Na^+$).

Most effective taken with meals and at bedtime. Consider laxative Px*.

▼AMFEBUTAMONE see Buproprion; adjunct to smoking cessation.

AMILORIDE
K$^+$-sparing diuretic (weak): inhibits DCT Na$^+$ reabsorption and K$^+$ excretion.
Use: oedema (2° to HF, cirrhosis or ↑aldosterone), HTN (esp in conjunction with ↑K$^+$-wasting diuretics as combination preparations; see Co-amilofruse and Co-amilozide).
CI: ↑K$^+$, R
Caution: DM, P/B/E.
SE: ↑K$^+$, **GI upset**, **headache**, dry mouth, ↓BP (esp postural), ↓Na$^+$, rash, confusion. Rarely encephalopathy, hepatic/renal dysfunction.
Interactions: ↑s lithium levels.
Dose: 5–20 mg od (or divide into bd doses).
☠ Beware if on other drugs that ↑K$^+$, e.g. spironolactone, triamterene, ACE-i, angiotensin II antagonists and ciclosporin. Do not give oral K$^+$ supplements inc dietary salt tablets. ☠

AMINOPHYLLINE
Methylxanthine bronchodilator: as theophylline but ↑H$_2$O solubility (is mixed w ethylenediamine) and ↓hypersensitivity.
Use/Caution/SE/Monitor/Interactions: see Theophylline; also available iv for use in acute severe bronchospasm; see pp. 183–4.
☠ NB: has many important interactions and can ⇒ arrhythmias (use cardiac monitor). ☠
Dose: po: 100–300 mg tds/qds. MR preparation (Phyllocontin Continus) ⇒ ↓SEs, has different doses at 225–450 mg bd (or 350–700 mg bd if Forte tablets – for smokers and others with short t$_{1/2}$). *If on a particular brand, ensure this is prescribed as they have different pharmacokinetics.*

iv: load* with 5 mg/kg (usually = 250–500 mg) over 20 min, then 0.5 mg/kg/h ivi, then adjusted to keep plasma levels at 10–20 mg/l (= 55–110 μmol/l). Omit loading dose* if patient not detoriorating.

☠ If already taking maintenance po aminophylline/theophylline, omit loading dose* and check levels ASAP to guide dosing. ☠

AMIODARONE

Class III antiarrhythmic: ↑s refractory period of conducting system (with limited myocardial depression).

Use: all tachyarrhythmias: paroxysmal SVT, AF, atrial flutter, nodal tachycardias, VT. Also in CPR/peri-arrest arrhythmias.

CI: ↓HR, sinoatrial HB, SAN disease, severe conduction disturbance w/o pacemaker, Hx of thyroid disease/iodine sensitivity, **P/B**.

Caution: porphyria, L/R/H/E.

SE: *Acute:* **N&V** (dose-dependent), **↓HR/BP**. *Chronic:* rarely but seriously **↑or↓T₄, interstitial lung disease** (e.g. fibrosis, *but reversible if caught early*), **hepatotoxicity**, **conduction disturbances** (esp ↓HR). *Common:* **malaise**, **fatigue**, headache, photosensitive skin (rarely 'grey-slate'), corneal deposits, optic neuritis (rare but can ↓vision), peripheral neuropathy, blood disorders, hypersensitivity.

Monitor: TFTs, LFTs (do baseline CXR and watch for ↑SOB/alveolitis).

Warn: avoid sunlight/use sunscreen.

Interactions: ↑s fx of phenytoin and digoxin. Many class I antiarrhythmics, antipsychotics, TCAs, co-trimoxazole, antimalarials, nelfinavir, ritonavir ⇒ ↑risk of ventricular arrhythmias. Verapamil, diltiazem and β-blockers ⇒ ↑risk of ↓HR and HB **W+**.

Dose: **po:** load with 200 mg tds in 1st wk, bd in 2nd wk, od from 3rd wk onwards (long $t_{1/2}$: months before steady plasma concentration); **iv:** (extreme emergencies only) 150–300 mg in 10–20 ml 5% glucose over ≥3 min (do not repeat for ≥15 min); **ivi:** 5 mg/kg over 20–120 min (max 1.2 g/day).

For use in cardiac arrest, NCT, BCT and AF, see ALS protocols in inside covers of this book.

L/R/H = **L**iver, **R**enal and **H**eart failure (full key see p. x)

☠ iv doses: give via central line (if no time for insertion, give via largest Venflon possible) with ECG monitoring. Avoid giving if severe respiratory failure or ↓BP (unless caused by arrhythmia) as can worsen. Avoid iv boluses if CCF/cardiomyopathy. ☠

AMITRIPTYLINE
Tricyclic antidepressant: blocks reuptake of NA (and 5-HT).
Use: depression[1] (esp if sedation beneficial), neuropathic pain[2].
CI: recent MI (w/in 3 months), arrhythmias (esp HB), mania, **L** (if severe).
Caution: cardiac/thyroid disease, epilepsy*, glaucoma (angle closure), phaeo, porphyria, anaesthesia. Also Hx of mania, psychosis or urinary retention, **H/P/B/E**.
SE: antimuscarinic fx (see p. 174), **cardiac fx** (arrhythmias, HB, ↑HR, postural ↓BP, dizziness, syncope: **dangerous in OD**), ↑Wt, **sedation**** (often ⇒ 'hangover'), seizures*, movement disorders. Rarely mania, fever, blood disorders, hypersensitivity, ΔLFTs, ↓Na⁺ (esp in elderly), neuroleptic malignant syndrome.
Warn: may impair driving**.
Interactions: ☠**MAOIs** ⇒ HTN and CNS excitation.☠ Levels ↑d by SSRIs, phenothiazines and cimetidine. ↑Risk of arrhythmias with **amiodarone**, pimozide, thioridazine and some class I antiarrhythmics. ↑s sedative fx of alcohol.
Dose: 75–200 mg nocte (or divided doses)[1]; 10–20 mg ↑ing to 75 mg nocte[2].

AMLODIPINE/ISTIN
Ca⁺⁺ channel blocker (dihydropyridine): as nifedipine, but ⇒ no ↓contractility or ↑HF.
Use: HTN, angina (esp 'Prinzmetal's' = coronary vasospasm).
CI: ACS, cardiogenic shock, aortic stenosis (unless mild), **P/B**.
Caution: L.
SE/Interactions: as nifedipine.
Dose: 5–10 mg od po.

AMOXICILLIN

Broad-spectrum penicillin. Similar to ampicillin but with ↑gastric absorption.

Use: mild pneumonias[1] (esp community-acquired), endocarditis Px, ENT/dental infections. *Often used with clavulanic acid as co-amoxiclav.*

CI/Caution/SE: see Ampicillin.

Dose: 500–1000 mg tds po/iv[1] (higher doses can be given according to indication[BNF]).

AMPICILLIN

Broad-spectrum penicillin for iv use: has ↓GI absorption cf amoxicillin, which is preferred po.

Use: Meningitis (esp *Listeria*; see p. 135)[1], Px preoperative or for endocarditis during invasive procedures if valve lesions/prostheses, respiratory tract/ENT infections (esp community-acquired pneumonia dt *Haemophilus influenzae* or *Streptococcus pneumoniae*), UTIs (not for blind Rx, as *Escherichia coli* often resistant).

CI: penicillin hypersensitivity.

Caution: EBV/CMV infections, ALL, CLL (all ↑risk of rash), R.

SE: rash* (erythematous, maculopapular: often does not reflect true allergy), **N&V&D** (rarely AAC), **hypersensitivity**, CNS/blood disorders.

Dose: 2 g 4-hourly ivi[1]; most other indications 0.25–1 g qds po/im/iv[BNF].

ANTABUSE see Disulfiram; adjunct to alcohol withdrawal.

APRACLONIDINE/IOPIDINE

Topical (ocular) α_2 agonist: ↓s aqueous humour production ∴ ↓s IOP.

Use: glaucoma: short-term Rx of severe cases.

CI: cardiovascular disease (severe or uncontrolled – inc Hx of).

Caution: IHD, vasovagal attacks, cerebrovascular disease, depression, R/H/P/B.

L/R/H = Liver, **Renal** and **Heart** failure (full key see p. x)

SE: dry mouth, taste Δ, local pruritus/discomfort (oedema), headache, asthenia, dry nose. Systemic fx can occur (see Clonidine).
Dose: 1 drop tds of 0.5% solution (1% available for perioperative specialist use).

ASACOL see Mesalazine: 'new' aminosalicylate for UC with ↓SEs. Available po (3–6 tablets of 400 mg per day in divided doses) or as foam enemas (1–2 g daily).

ASPIRIN

NSAID. Inhibits COX-1 and COX-2. Also anti-Pt action by inhibiting thromboxane A2.
Use: analgesic/anti-inflammatory/antipyrexial[1], IHD and thromboembolic CVA Px[2] and acute Rx[3].
CI: <16 years old (⇒ Reye's syndrome: liver and brain damage), **GI ulcers** (active or PHx of), bleeding disorders, gout, hypersensitivity (to any NSAID), **B**.
Caution: asthma, uncontrolled HTN, any allergic disease*, G6PD deficiency, dehydration, **L/R/P/E**.
SE: bleeding (esp GI: ↑↑risk if also anticoagulated)**. Rarely ARF, blood disorders, hypersensitivity* (anaphylaxis, bronchospasm, skin reactions), ototoxic in OD.
Interactions. W ↑ (↑anticoagulant fx, has additive fx on risk of bleeding)**.
Dose: 300–900 mg 4–6-hourly (max 4 g/day)[1], 75 mg od[2], 300 mg stat[3].
Stop 7 days before surgery if significant bleeding is expected. If cardiac surgery or patient has unstable angina, consider continuing.

ATENOLOL

β-blocker: (mildly) cardioselective* ($\beta_1 > \beta_2$), ↑H_2O solubility ∴ ↓central fx** and ↑renal excretion***.
Use: HTN[1], angina[2], MI (w/in 12 h as early intervention)[3], arrhythmias[4].

CI/SE: see Propranolol, but ⇒ ↓bronchospasm* (still avoid in asthma/COPD unless no other choice) and ↓sleep disturbance/nightmares**.
Dose: 25–50 mg od po[1]; 50 mg bd po[2]; 5 mg iv over 5 min then 50 mg po 15 min later then start 50 mg bd 12 h later[3]; 25–50 mg bd po[4] (if acute arrhythmia give iv[BNF]). Consider ↓ing dose in RF***.

ATORVASTATIN/LIPITOR
HMG-CoA reductase inhibitor.
Use/CI/Caution/SE: see Simvastatin.
Dose: 10 mg nocte (↑if necessary to 40 mg – max 80 mg).

iv ATROPINE (SULPHATE)
Muscarinic antagonist: blocks vagal SAN and AVN stimulation, bronchodilates and ↓s oropharyngeal secretions.
Use: severe ↓HR (see algorithm in inside front cover) or HB[1], CPR[2] (see ALS universal algorithm in inside back cover), organophosphate/anticholinesterase* OD/poisoning[3].
CI: (do not apply if life threatening condition/CPR!): glaucoma (angle closure), MG (unless xs anticholinesterase Rx, when atropine is indicated*), paralytic ileus, pyloric stenosis, ↑prostate.
Caution: Down's syndrome, gastro-oesophageal reflux, diarrhoea, UC, acute MI, HTN, ↑HR (esp 2° to ↑T_4, cardiac insufficiency or surgery), pyrexia, **P/B/E**.
SE: transient ↓HR (followed by ↑HR, palpitations, arrhythmias), **antimuscarinic fx** (see p. 174), N&V, confusion (esp in elderly), dizziness.
Dose: 0.3–1.0 mg iv[1], 3 mg iv[2] (if no iv access, give 6 mg with 10 ml saline via endotracheal tube), 2 mg im/iv every 10–30 min[3] (every 5 min in severe cases up to max 100 mg in 1st 24 h, until symptomatic response: skin flushes and dries, pupils dilate, HR ↑s).

ATROVENT see Ipratropium

AUGMENTIN see Co-amoxiclav (amoxicillin + clavulanic acid) 375 or 625 mg tds po (1.2 g tds iv).

AZATHIOPRINE

Antiproliferative immunosuppressant: inhibits purine-salvage pathways.

Use: prevention of transplant rejection, autoimmune disease (mostly as steroid-sparing agent, except as maintenance Rx for SLE and vasculitis).

CI: hypersensitivity (to azathioprine *or mercaptopurine*).

Caution: L/R/P/E.

SE: myelosuppression (dose-dependent, $\Rightarrow$ $\uparrow$infections, esp HZV), **hepatotoxicity**, **hypersensitivity reactions** (inc interstitial nephritis: *stop drug!*), **N&V&D** (esp initially), pancreatitis. Rarely cholestasis, pancreatitism, alopecia, pneumonitis, risk of neoplasia.

Monitor: FBC, LFTs.

Interactions: fx $\uparrow$ by **allopurinol** & ACE-i ($\Rightarrow$ $\uparrow$myelosuppression).

Dose: 1–5 mg/kg daily^{BNF} (preferably po as iv is very irritant).

☠ Before starting Rx, screen for common gene defect of the enzyme TPMT (which metabolises azathioprine): if homozygote for defect avoid azathioprine; if heterozygote, $\downarrow$dose. ☠

▼AZOPT see Brinzolamide

AZT see Zidovudine

BACLOFEN

Skeletal muscle relaxant: $\downarrow$s spinal reflexes, general CNS inhibition at $\uparrow$doses.

Use: spasticity, if chronic/severe, (esp 2° to MS or cord pathology).

CI: PU.

Caution: Ψ disorders, epilepsy, DM, hypertonic bladder sphincter, respiratory/cerebrovascular disease, R/P/E.

SE: sedation, $\downarrow$**muscle tone**, GI upset. Others rare: $\uparrow$spasticity (*stop drug!*), multiple neuro-Ψ symptoms, cardiac/hepatic/respiratory dysfunction.

Warn: may ↓skilled tasks (esp driving), ↑s fx of alcohol.
Dose: 5 mg tds po, ↑ to max of 100 mg/day. In severe cases, can give by intrathecal pump (see BNF/product literature).

Stop gradually over ⩾1–2 weeks to avoid withdrawal symptoms (hyperactivity, ↑spasticity, Ψ reactions, fits, autonomic dysfunction).

BACTROBAN see Mupirocin; topical antibiotic (esp for nasal MRSA). See local policy for infection control.

BALSALAZIDE
'New' aminosalicylate: prodrug of 5-ASA (↓sulphonamide SEs cf sulfasalazine).
Use/CI/Caution/SE: as mesalazine.
Dose: 2.25 g tds in acute attack, ↓ing to 1.5 g bd once in remission – adjust according to response.

BECLOFORTE see Beclometasone (high dose at 250 µg/puff).

BECLOMETASONE
Inh corticosteroid: ↓s airway oedema and mucous secretions.
Use: chronic asthma not controlled by short-acting β_2 agonists alone (start at step 2 of BTS guidelines; see p. 139).
Caution: TB (inc quiescent).
SE: oral candidiasis ($2°$ to immunosuppression: ↓d by rinsing mouth with H_2O after use), **hoarse voice**. Rarely glaucoma, hypersensitivity. ↑Doses may ⇒ adrenal suppression, ↓bone density, ↓growth (controversial).
Dose: 200–2000 µg daily inh (normally start at 200 µg bd). Use high-dose inhaler if daily requirements are >800 µg^{BNF}.

Rarely ⇒ paradoxical bronchospasm: can be prevented by switching from aerosol to dry powder forms or by using inh β_2 agonists.

BECOTIDE see Beclometasone (50, 100 or 200 µg/puff).

L/R/H = Liver, Renal and Heart failure (full key see p. x)

BENDROFLUMETHIAZIDE (previously BENDROFLUAZIDE)

Thiazide diuretic: $\downarrow$s Na^+ (and Cl^-) reabsorbtion from DCT $\Rightarrow Na^+$ and H_2O loss and stimulates K^+ excretion.

Use: oedema[1] (2° to HF or low–protein states), HTN[2] (in short term by $\downarrow$ing fluid volume and CO; in long term by $\downarrow$ing TPR), Px against renal stones in hypercalciuria[3].

CI: $\downarrow K^+$ (refractory to Rx), $\downarrow Na^+$, $\uparrow Ca^{++}$, Addison's disease, $\uparrow$urate (if symptoms), **L/R** (if either severe, otherwise caution).

Caution: porphyria, and can worsen gout, DM or SLE, P/B/E.

SE: dehydration (esp in elderly), $\downarrow$**BP** (esp postural), $\downarrow K^+$, GI upset, **impotence**, $\downarrow Na^+$, alkalosis (with $\downarrow Cl^-$), $\downarrow Mg^{++}$, $\uparrow Ca^{++}$, $\uparrow$urate/gout, $\uparrow$glucose, Δlipid metabolism (esp $\uparrow$cholesterol), rash, photosensitivity, blood disorders (inc $\downarrow$Pt, $\downarrow$NØ), pancreatitis, intrahepatic cholestasis, hyper-sensitivity reactions (inc severe respiratory and skin reactions).

Dose: initially 5–10 mg mane po[1] (if possible, then $\downarrow$frequency rather than amount of dose); 2.5 mg od po[2,3] (no real benefit from $\uparrow$doses).

BENZYLPENICILLIN

Penicillin with poor po absorption ∴ only given im/iv: used mostly against streptococcal (esp *S. pneumoniae*) and neisserial (esp *N. gonorrhoeae*, *N. meningitidis*) infections.

Use: severe skin infections (esp cellulitis, wound infections, gas gangrene) in conjunction with other agents (see p. 136), meningitis, endocarditis, ENT infections.

CI: penicillin hypersensitivity.

Caution: R*.

SE: hypersensitivity (inc fever, arthralgia, rashes, urticaria, angioedema, anaphylaxis, serum sickness-like reactions, haemolytic $\downarrow$Hb, interstitial nephritis), **diarrhoea** (rarely AAC). Rarely blood disorders ($\downarrow$Pt, $\downarrow$NØ, coagulation disorders), CNS toxicity (inc convulsions, esp at $\uparrow$doses or if RF*).

Dose: 1.2 g qds iv (or im/ivi). If very severe, give 2.4 g every 4 h (only as iv/ivi).

BETAGAN see Levobunolol 0.5% (β-blocker): eye drops for glaucoma.

BETAHISTINE/SERC

Histamine analogue: ↑s middle-ear microcirculation
⇒ ↓endolymphatic pressure.
Use: Ménière's disease (if tinnitus, vertigo or hearing loss).
CI: phaeo.
Caution: asthma, Hx of PU, P/B.
SE: GI upset. Rarely headache, rash, pruritus.
Dose: 16 mg tds po (maintenance normally 24–48 mg/day).

BETAMETHASONE CREAM (0.1%)

'Potent' strength topical corticosteroid (rarely used as weaker 0.05% or 0.025% preparations).

BETNOVATE see Betamethasone cream 0.1% (potent strength). Also available as Betnovate RD (moderate strength) 0.025% preparation.

BEZAFIBRATE

Fibrate (lipid-lowering): ⇒ ↓TG, ↓LDL, ↑HDL by stimulating lipoprotein lipase (⇒ ↓conversion of VLDL/TG to LDL and ⇒ ↑LDL clearance from circulation). Also ⇒ (mild) ↓cholesterol.
Use: hyperlipidaemias (esp if ↑TG ∴ types IIa/b, III, IV, V).
CI: gallbladder disease, PBC, ↓albumin (esp nephrotic syndrome), **L** (if severe), P/B.
Caution: ↓T₄ (needs to be corrected), R*.
SE: GI upset, ↑**gallstones, myositis** (rarer but important: ↑risk if RF*). Also impotence, rash (inc pruritus, urticaria), headache. Rarer: dizziness, vertigo, fatigue, hair loss, blood disorders (↓Hb, ↓WCC, ↓Pt).
Interactions: statins ↑risk of myositis, can ↑renal toxicity of ciclosporin. **W+**.
Dose: 200 mg tds po (after food). MR 400 mg od preps availableBNF.

BICARBONATE see Sodium bicarbonate

BISOPROLOL

β-blocker, cardioselective ($β_1 > β_2$).
Use: HTN[1], angina[2], HF[3].
CI/Caution/SE/Interactions: as propranolol, but also CI in HF
needing inotropes or if SAN block; caution if psoriasis.
Dose: 10 mg od po[1,2] (maintenance 5–20 mg od); initially 1.25 mg
od po[3] (↑ing slowly to max 10 mg od).
Consider ↓ing doses in RF and LF.

BOWEL PREPARATIONS

Bowel-cleansing solutions for preparation for GI surgery/Ix.
CI: GI obstruction/ulceration/perforation, ileus, gastric retention,
toxic megacolon/colitis, **H**.
Caution: UC, DM, heart disease, reflux oesophagitis, ↑risk of
regurgitation/aspiration (e.g. ↓swallow or ↓GCS), **R/P**.
SE: nausea, bloating, abdominal pains, vomiting.
Dose: see Citramag, Fleet, Klean-prep, Picolax.

BRICANYL see Terbutaline (inh $β_2$ agonist for asthma). Various
delivery devices available[BNF].

BRIMONIDINE EYE DROPS/ALPHAGAN

Topical $α_2$ agonist: ↓s aqueous humour production ∴ ↓s IOP.
Use: open-angle glaucoma, ocular HTN (2nd-line if β-blocker drops
are unsuitable or control IOP inadequately).
Caution: postural ↓BP, Raynaud's, cardiovascular disease (esp
IHD), cerebral insufficiency, depression, **P/B/R/L**.
SE: sedation, headache, blurred vision, dry mouth/nose, **local
reactions** (esp discomfort, pruritus, hyperaemia, follicular
conjunctivitis). Rarely HTN, palpitations, depression,
hypersensitivity.
Dose: 1 drop bd of 0.2% solution.

▼BRINZOLAMIDE/AZOPT

Topical carbonic anhydrase inhibitor for glaucoma. Similar to
dorzolamide (↓s aqueous humour production).
Dose: 1 drop bd/tds (of 10 mg/ml solution).

BROMOCRIPTINE

DA agonist.
Use: parkinsonism if L-dopa insufficient/not tolerated. Also
endocrine disorders if prolactin or growth hormone related
(DA ⇒ ↓pituitary release of these hormones).
CI: toxaemia of pregnancy, hypersensitivity to ergot alkaloids. Also
HTN/IHD postpartum or in puerperium.
Caution: cardiovascular disease, porphyria, Raynaud's disease,
serious Ψ disorders (esp psychosis), P/B.
SE: GI upset, postural ↓BP (esp initially and if ↑alcohol intake),
behavioural Δs (confusional states, Ψ disorders). Rarely
but seriously **fibrosis***: pulmonary**, cardiac, retroperitoneal***
(can ⇒ ARF).
Monitor: ESR*, U&Es***, CXR**.
Dose: 1–30 mg/day[BNF].

BUCCASTEM Prochlorperazine (antiemetic) buccal tablets:
absorbed rapidly from under top lip ∴ do not need to be swallowed
and retained in stomach for absorption if N&V.
Dose: 3–6 mg bd.

BUDESONIDE

Inh corticosteroid similar to beclometasone but stronger
(approximately double the strength per microgram).
Dose: 200–800 μg bd inh (aerosol or powder) or 1–2 mg bd neb.

BUMETANIDE

Loop diuretic.
Use/CI/Caution/SE: as furosemide; also can ⇒ myalgia at ↑doses.
Dose: 1 mg mane po (500 μg may suffice in elderly), ↑ing if
required (5 mg/24 h usually sufficient; ↑by adding a lunchtime dose,

then ↑ing each dose). 1–2 mg im/iv (repeat after 20 min if required).
2–5 mg ivi over 30–60 min.

NB: give iv in severe oedema (as bowel is often also oedematous
∴ ↓po absorption).

▼BUPROPION (= AMFEBUTAMONE)/ZYBAN

NA and to lesser extent DA reuptake inhibitor (NDRI) developed as
antidepressant, but also ↑s success of giving up smoking.
Use: (adjunct to) smoking cessation[NICE].
CI: CNS tumour, acute alcohol/benzodiazepine withdrawal, Hx of
seizures*, eating disorders, bipolar disorder, **P/B**.
Caution: if ↑risk of seizures*: alcohol abuse, Hx of head trauma
and DM, **L/R/E**.
SE: seizures*, insomnia (and other CNS reactions, e.g. anxiety,
agitation, depression, headaches, tremor, dizziness). Also ↑HR,
AV block, ↑ or ↓BP**, hypersensitivity (inc severe skin reactions),
GI upset, ↑Wt, mild antimuscarinic fx (esp **dry mouth**; see p. 174
for others).
Monitor: BP**.
Interactions: ↓P450 ∴ many interactions, but importantly **CNS
drugs, esp if ↓seizure threshold***, e.g. antidepressants,
antimalarials, antipsychotics, quinolones, sedating antihistamines,
systemic corticosteroids, theophyllines, tramadol. Ritonavir
⇒ ↑toxic fx.
Dose: 150 mg od for 6 days then 150 mg bd for max 9 wks (↓dose
in elderly[BNF]).

BURINEX Bumetanide 1-mg tablets. Also available as K⁺-
conserving preparations: Burinex A (1 mg bumetanide + 5 mg
amiloride) and Burinex K (0.5 mg bumetanide + 7.7 mmol K⁺).

BUSCOPAN see Hyoscine butylbromide; GI antispasmodic.

CACIT see Calcium carbonate

CACIT D3 Calcium carbonate + low-dose vitamin D_3
(cholecalciferol).

Use: Px of vitamin D deficiency.
Dose: 1 tablet od (= 12.6 mmol Ca^{++} + 11 μg cholecalciferol).

CALCICHEW see Calcium carbonate

CALCICHEW D3 Calcium carbonate + low–dose vitamin D_3 (cholecalciferol).
Use: Px of vitamin D deficiency.
Dose: 1 tablet od (= 12.6 mmol Ca^{++} + 5 μg cholecalciferol (or 10 μg in 'forte' preparations)).

CALCITONIN

Synthetic hormone (normally produced by C cells of thyroid): binds to specific osteoclast receptors ⇒ ↓resorption of bone and ↓Ca^{++}. Its fx are specific to abnormal (high-turnover) bone.
Use: ↑Ca^{++} (esp dt malignancy; also ↓s bone metastases pain), Paget's disease (↓s pain and neurological symptoms, e.g. deafness), rarely for Px/Rx of postmenopausal osteoporosis.
Caution: Hx of *any* allergy, R/H/P/B.
SE: GI upset (esp N&V), **flushing**, ↑**urinary frequency**, taste and sensory Δ, hypersensitivity (inc anaphylaxis), local inflammation.
Dose: see BNF/product literature.

CALCIUM CARBONATE

Use: osteoporosis, ↓Ca^{++}, ↑PO_4 (esp 2° to RF; binds PO_4 in gut ⇒ ↓absorption).
CI: ↑Ca^{++} (in serum or urine).
Caution: sarcoid, R.
Dose: according to requirements, up to 40 mmol/day in osteoporosis if ↓dietary intake, e.g. Calcichew (standard 12.6-mmol or 'forte' 25-mmol tablets), Cacit (12.6-mmol tablets), Calcium 500 (12.5-mmol tablets) or Adcal (15-mmol tablets).

L/R/H = **L**iver, **R**enal and **H**eart failure (full key see p. x)

CALCIUM CHLORIDE

Ca^{++} for emergency iv use: mostly CPR as $\Rightarrow$ $\uparrow$venous irritation cf calcium gluconate (can also be used for severe $\downarrow Ca^{++}$ or $\uparrow K^+$).
Dose: available as syringes of 10 ml of 10% solution (= total of 6.8 mmol Ca^{++}). Give iv no quicker than 1 ml/min (otherwise can $\Rightarrow$ arrhythmias) according to indication and clinical/electrolyte response.
e.g. Min-i-jet: often in crash trolleys if iv Ca^{++} needed urgently.

CALCIUM + ERGOCALCIFEROL tablets of 2.4 mmol Ca^{++} + low-dose (10 µg) ergocalciferol (= calciferol = vitamin D_2).
Use: Px of vitamin D deficiency.
CI/Caution/SE: see ergocalciferol.
Dose: 1 tablet od.

CALCIUM GLUCONATE

iv preparation of Ca^{++} (also available po, but used rarely).
Use: $\downarrow Ca^{++}$ (if severe)[1], $\uparrow K^+$ ($\downarrow$s arrhythmias: 'cardioprotective', see p. 190)[2], $\uparrow Mg^{++}$.
Dose: 10 ml of 10% iv over 2 min (= total of 2.2 mmol Ca^{++})[1,2], repeating if necessary according to clinical and electrolyte response; consider following with ivi[1].

CALCIUM RESONIUM

Polystyrene sulphonate ion-exchange resin.
Use: mild/moderate $\uparrow K^+$.
CI: obstructive bowel disease, diseases likely to $\uparrow Ca^{++}$ (hyper-parathyroidism, multiple myeloma, sarcoid, metastatic cancer).
Caution: P/B.
SE: GI upset (esp constipation; often need Px of 10–20 ml lactulose), $\downarrow K^+$, $\uparrow Ca^{++}$ and Na^+ retention.
Dose: 15 g tds/qds po. NB: takes 24–48 h to work. Also available as 30-g enemas (rarely $\Rightarrow$ rectal ulceration and colonic necrosis: needs cleansing enema first and washout afterwards; see product literature).

CALPOL Paracetamol (paediatric) suspension.

Dose: according to age; all doses can be given up to max frequency qds (min dose spacing = 4 h): 3 months–1 year 60–120 mg, 1–5 years 120–250 mg, 6–12 years 250–500 mg, >12 years 500–1000 mg (= adult dose).

Two strengths available: 'standard' (120 mg/5 ml) and '6 plus' (250 mg/5 ml).

CANDESARTAN/AMIAS

Angiotensin II antagonist.
Use: HTN.
CI: cholestasis, **P/B**.
Caution/SE/Interactions: see Losartan.
Dose: initially 2–4 mg od, ↑ing if necessary to max of 16 mg od.

CANESTEN Clotrimazole 1% cream: antifungal, esp for vaginal candida infections (thrush). Also available as powder, solution and spray for hairy areas.
Dose: apply bd/tds.

CAPTOPRIL

ACE inhibitor: short-acting; largely replaced by longer-acting (od) ACEi drugs.
Use: HTN, HF, post-MI, and diabetic nephropathy (i.e. consistent proteinuria).
CI: renovascular disease* (known or suspected bilateral RAS), angioedema/other hypersensitivity 2° to ACEi, porphyria, **P**.
Caution: symptomatic aortic stenosis, Hx of idiopathic or hereditary angioedema, **R/B/E**.
SE: ↓**BP** (esp with 1st dose, if HF, dehydrated or on diuretics, dialysis or ↓Na⁺ diet ∴ *take at night*), **RF***, **dry cough**, ↑K⁺, **hypersensitivity** (esp rashes and **angioedema**), Δ taste, upper respiratory tract symptoms (inc sore throat/sinusitis/rhinitis), GI upset, Δ LFTs (rarely cholestatic jaundice/hepatitis), pancreatitis, blood disorders, many nonspecific neurological symptoms.

Monitor: U&Es, esp baseline and *2 wks after starting**.
Interactions: fx ↓d by NSAIDs (also ⇒ ↑risk RF*). Diuretics
⇒ risk of ↓BP. ↑s fx of lithium.
Dose: 6.25–75 mg bd po[BNF].

☠Beware if on other drugs that ↑K+, e.g. amiloride, spironolactone, triamterene, angiotensin II antagonists and ciclosporin.
Do not give with oral K+ supplements – inc dietary salt
substitutes. ☠

CARBAMAZEPINE/TEGRETOL

Antiepileptic, mood stabiliser, analgesic; ↓s synaptic transmission.
Use: epilepsy[1], bipolar disorder[2] (2nd-line), neuralgia[3] (esp
post-herpetic, trigeminal and DM-related).
CI: unpaced AV conduction dfx, Hx of BM suppression, porphyria .
Caution: cardiac disease, Hx skin disorders or haematological drug
reactions, glaucoma, **L/R, P** (⇒ neural tube dfx* ∴ ⇒ folate Px and
screen for dfx), **B**.
Dose-related SEs: dizziness, vertigo, ataxia, visual Δ
(esp double vision): control by ↓ing dose, Δ dose times/
spacing or use of MR preparations**. **Other SEs: skin
reactions, blood disorders** (esp ↓WCC*** – often transient,
esp initially), **GI upset, ↓Na+** (inc SIADH), **drowsiness**, HF,
arrhythmias, AV block, pulmonary hypersensitivity. Many rarer
SEs[BNF].
Monitor: serum levels (optimum therapeutic range = 4–12 mg/l),
U&Es, LFTs, FBC***.
Warn: driving may be impaired, and watch for signs of liver/skin/
haematological disease.
Interactions: ↑P450 ∴ many; most importantly, fx are ↑d by
erythromycin/clarithromycin, isoniazid, verapamil and diltiazem;
and it ↓s fx of **OCP** (NB: *carbamazepine is teratogenic!**),
corticosteroids, other antiepileptics (NB: *can also autoinduce!*)
and **W−**.
Dose: initially 100–200 mg od/bd (↑slowly to max of 1.6 g/day[2,3] or
2 g/day[1]). (MR forms** available[BNF])

CARBIMAZOLE

Thionamide anti-thyroid: peroxidase inhibitor; stops $I^- \Rightarrow I_2$ and $\therefore \downarrow$s T_3/T_4 production. ?Also immunosuppressive fx.

Use: $\uparrow T_4$.

Caution: L, P/B (can cause fetal/neonatal goitre/$\downarrow T_4$ $\therefore$ use min dose to control symptoms and monitor neonatal development closely – 'block-and-replace' regimen $\therefore$ not suitable).

SE: hypersensitivity: rash and **pruritus** (if symptoms not tolerated or not eased by antihistamines, switch to propylthiouracil), fever, arthralgia. Also GI disturbance (esp nausea), headache. Rarely hepatic dysfunction, alopecia, blood disorders – esp **agranulocytosis*** (0.5%) and $\downarrow$WCC (often transient and benign).

Dose: 15–60 mg od ($\downarrow$dose once euthyroid; maintenance dose usually 5–15 mg od, unless on block-and-replace regimen, where $\uparrow$d doses are maintained). *Normally give for only 12–18 months.* Remission often occurs; if not, other Rx (e.g. surgery/radioiodine) may be needed.

☠**Agranulocytosis:** warn patient to report immediately signs/symptoms of infection (esp sore throat, but also fever, malaise, mouth ulcers, bruising and nonspecific illness). If suspect infection, do FBC (routine screening unhelpful as can occur rapidly). Stop drug if clinical or laboratory evidence of $\downarrow$NØ*.☠

▼CARVEDILOL

β-blocker: nonselective but also blocks α_1 $\therefore$ $\Rightarrow$ arterial vasodilation.

Use: HF[1] (if stable). Less commonly for angina[2] and HTN[3].

CI/Caution: as propranolol, plus **L**, and avoid in HF if severe/needs iv inotropes.

SE: as propranolol, but worse postural $\downarrow$BP.

Dose: initially 3.125 mg bd[1] ($\uparrow$ing slowly to max of 25–50 mg bd); initially 12.5 mg bd[2]/od[3] (can $\uparrow$ to 50 mg/day).

CEFACLOR

Oral 2nd-generation cephalosporin.

Use: mild respiratory infections, UTIs, external infections (skin/soft-tissue infections, sinusitis, otitis media), esp in pregnancy* (safer than other drugs) or dt *H. influenzae*.

CI: cephalosporin hypersensitivity, porphyria.

Caution: penicillin hypersensitivity (10% also allergic to cephalosporins), R (no dose adjustment required – but can be necessary for other cephalosporins[BNF]), P/B (but appropriate to use*).

SE: GI upset (esp N&D, rarely AAC), **allergy** (anaphylaxis, fever, arthralgia, skin reactions (inc severe)), **ARF**, **interstitial nephritis** (reversible), hepatic dysfunction, blood disorders, CNS disturbance (inc headache).

Dose: 250 mg tds po (max 4 g/day).

Can ⇒ false-positive urinary glucose and Coombs' test (as can all cephalosporins).

CEFALEXIN

Oral 1st-generation cephalosporin.

Use/CI/Caution/SE: see Cefaclor.

Dose: 250 mg qds or 500 mg bd/tds po (max 6 g/day). For Px of UTI, give 125 mg po nocte.

CEFOTAXIME

Parenteral 3rd-generation cephalosporin.

Use: severe infections, esp meningitis and sepsis 2° to hospital-acquired pneumonia, UTI, pyelonephritis, soft-tissue infections.

CI/Caution/SE: see Cefaclor.

Dose: 1 g bd im/iv/ivi (↑ing to max of 3 g qds if needed).

CEFRADINE

Oral or parenteral 1st-generation cephalosporin.

Use: as cefaclor, plus preoperative Px[1].

CI/Caution/SE: see Cefaclor.

Dose: 1–2 g im/iv at induction[1]; otherwise 0.25–1 g qds po/im/iv/ivi, ↑ing to max of 8 g/day in very severe infections.

CEFTAZIDIME

Parenteral 3rd-generation cephalosporin: good against *Pseudomonas*.
Use: see Cefotaxime (often reserved for ITU setting).
CI/Caution/SE: see Cefaclor.
Dose: 1 g tds im/iv/ivi, ↑ing (with care in elderly) to 2 g tds iv
(not im, where max single dose is 1 g) if life-threatening,
e.g. meningitis, immunocompromised.

CEFTRIAXONE

Parenteral 3rd-generation cephalosporin.
Use: as cefotaxime, plus preoperative Px[1].
CI/Caution/SE: as cefaclor, plus **L** (if coexistent RF), **R** (if severe),
caution if dehydrated, young or immobile (can precipitate in urine
or gallbladder). Rarely ⇒ pancreatitis and ↑PT.
Dose: 1 g od im/iv/ivi (max 4 g/day); 1–2 g im/iv/ivi at induction[1].
Max im dose = 1 g per site; if total >1 g, give at divided sites.

CEFUROXIME

Parenteral and oral 2nd-generation cephalosporin: good for some
Gram-negative infections (*H. influenzae*, *N. gonorrhoeae*) and better
than 3rd-generation cephalosporins for Gram-positive infections
(esp *S. aureus*).
Use: *po:* respiratory infections[1], UTIs[2], pyelonephritis[3]; *iv:* severe
infections[4], preoperative Px[5].
CI/Caution/SE: see Cefaclor.
Dose: 250–500 mg bd po[1]; 125 mg bd po[2]; 250 mg bd po[3];
750 mg tds/qds iv/im[4] (1.5 g tds/qds iv in very severe infections);
1.5 g iv at induction (+750 mg iv/im tds for 24 h if high-risk
procedure)[5].

CELECOXIB/CELEBREX

NSAID with selective inhibition of COX-2 ∴ ↓GI SEs
(COX-1-mediated). *Provides no Px against ischaemic events*
(unlike aspirin).
Use: osteoarthritis/rheumatoid arthritis symptomatic relief[NICE].

CI: Active PU/GI bleeding, hypersensitivity to any NSAID (inc asthma, angioedema, urticaria, acute rhinitis), *sulphonamide* hypersensitivity, IBD, **L/R/H** (if severe – otherwise/caution) **P/B**.
Caution: Hx of PU/GI bleeding, HTN, oedema (of any cause).
SE/Interactions: as ibuprofen, but ↓**GI ulceration/bleeding**. Also can ⇒ peripheral oedema (even if no predisposing cause), GI upset, HTN, back pain, headache, dizziness.
Dose: 100–200 mg bd po.

> NICE guidelines do not recommend routine use, or use if cardiovascular disease (where benefit lost if also taking aspirin). Only use if Hx of PU, GI bleeding/perforation or ↑risk of serious GI SEs (e.g. age >65 years, debilitated, on other medications w ↑risk of GI bleed, or have been on long-term Rx of unselective NSAIDs at max doses).

CEPH– see CEF–

CETIRIZINE/ZIRTEK

Non-sedating antihistamine: selectively inhibits peripheral H_1 receptors.
Use: allergy; symptomatic relief from (esp hay fever, urticaria).
CI: P/B.
Caution: epilepsy, R, L.
SE: mild antimuscarinic fx (see p. 174), very mild sedation, headache.
Warn: may impair driving.
Dose: 10 mg od (or 5 mg bd) po.

CHARCOAL

Binds and ↓s absorption of tablets/poisons.
Use: ODs (up to 1 h post-ingestion; longer if MR/SR preparations or antimuscarinic drugs. See p. 192).
Caution: corrosive poisons, ↓GI motility (can ⇒ obstruction), ↓GCS (risk of inhalation, unless endotracheal tube in situ).
Dose: 50 g (mix with 200 ml water). Give once for paracetamol, salicylates and TCAs. Repeated doses (every 4 h) often needed for

barbiturates, carbamazepine, phenytoin, digoxin, dapsone, paraquat, quinine, theophylline and MR/SR preparations.

CHLORAMPHENICOL

Broad-spectrum antibiotic: inhibits bacterial protein synthesis; very potent action, but SEs limit use.

Use: severe infections (esp *H. influenzae*) and rickettsiae (e.g. typhoid).
CI: porphyria **P/B**.
Caution: **L** (↓dose*), **R**.
SE: blood disorders (inc aplastic ↓Hb), neuritis (peripheral, optic), GI upset, hepatotoxicity, hypersensitivity, stomatitis, glossitis.
Monitor: FBC (and serum drug levels if LF*).
Interactions: ↑s fx of sulphonylureas and phenytoin. Phenobarbital ↓s its fx. **W+**.
Dose: 50 mg/kg/day in 4 divided doses iv (or rarely po), ↑ing to 100 mg/kg if life-threatening infection.

CHLORAMPHENICOL EYE DROPS

Topical preparation, with no significant systemic fx, for superficial bacterial eye infections.
Dose: 1 × 0.5% drop to affected eye(s) at least 2-hourly (↓once infection controlled, continue after healed for 48 h). Can give as 1% ointment applied tds/qds (or nocte only if taking drops in daytime as well).

CHLORDIAZEPOXIDE

Benzodiazepine, long-acting.
Use: anxiety (esp in alcohol withdrawal).
CI/Caution/SE: see Diazepam, plus **W–**.
Dose: 10 mg tds po, ↑ing if required to max of 100 mg/day. ↓dose in elderly, ↑dose if benzodiazepine-resistant or in initial Rx of alcohol withdrawal (see p. 147 for reducing regime).

CHLORHEXIDINE

Disinfectant mouthwash or solution for skin cleansing before invasive procedures and bladder washout.

CHLORMETHIAZOLE see Clomethiazole; used in alcohol withdrawal.

CHLOROQUINE

Antimalarial: inhibits protein synthesis and DNA/RNA polymerases.
Use: malaria Px (only as Rx if 'benign', i.e. non-*Falciparum* spp, which are often resistant).
Caution: G6PD deficiency, severe GI disorders, can worsen psoriasis and MG, neurological disorders (esp epilepsy*), L (avoid other hepatotoxic drugs), R/P.
SE: GI upset, headache (mild, transient), **visual Δ** (rarely retinopathy**), **seizures***, hypersensitivity/skin reactions (inc pigment Δs), hair loss. Rarely **BM suppression** and arrhythmias (common in OD).
Monitor: vision**.
Dose: *Px:* 300 mg once weekly *as base (specify on prescription: do not confuse with salt doses).* Used mostly in conjunction with other drugs, depending on local resistance patterns[BNF]. Rx: see p. 134.

CHLORPHEN(IR)AMINE/PIRITON

Sedating antihistamine: H_1 antagonist.
Use: allergies[1] (esp drug reactions, hay fever, urticaria), anaphylaxis[2] (inc blood transfusion reaction[3]).
CI: MAOI given w/in last 2 wks (↑s antimuscarinic fx).
Caution: pyloroduodenal obstruction, urinary retention (and ↑prostate), glaucoma, epilepsy, R/L/P/B.
SE: drowsiness (rarely paradoxical stimulation), **antimuscarinic** fx (esp dry mouth; see p. 174), GI upset, arrhythmias, ↓BP, skin and hypersensitivity reactions (inc bronchospasm, photosensitivity).
Warn: driving may be impaired.
Dose: 4 mg 4–6-hourly po[1]; 10 mg iv over 1 min[2] (can ↑iv dose to 20 mg), continuing for 24–48 h as Px against relapse (max 40 mg in 24 h); 10–20 mg sc[3].

CHLORPROMAZINE

Antipsychotic (phenothiazine) $\Rightarrow$ DA blockade (esp $D_{1\&3} > D_{2\&4}$).
Also blocks $5HT_{2A}$, histamine (H_1), adrenergic ($\alpha_{1>2}$) and muscarinic receptors.

Use: schizophrenia[1], acute sedation[2] (inc mania, severe anxiety, violent behaviour), intractable hiccups[3].

CI: CNS depression (inc coma), Hx of blood dyscrasias, severe cardiovascular disease.

Caution: Parkinson's disease, epilepsy, MG, phaeo, glaucoma (angle-closure), ↑prostate, severe respiratory disease, jaundice, blood disorders, predisposition to postural ↓BP, ↑or ↓temperature. Avoid direct sunlight (⇒ photosensitivity), **L/R/H/P/B/E**.

Class SE: sedation, extrapyramidal fx (see pp. 175–6), **antimuscarinic fx** (see p. 174), **seizures**, ↑**Wt**, ↓**BP** (esp postural), ECG Δs (↑QTc), arrhythmias, endocrine fx (menstrual Δs, galactorrhoea, gynaecomastia, sexual dysfunction), ΔLFTs/jaundice, blood disorders (inc agranulocytosis, ↓WCC), ↓ or ↑temperature (esp in elderly), rash/↑pigmentation, **neuroleptic malignant syndrome**.

Warn: avoid alcohol, ↓s skilled tasks (inc driving).

Interactions: fx ↑d by TCAs (esp antimuscarinic fx), lithium (esp extrapyramidal fx +/– neurotoxicity), cimetidine and β-blockers (esp arrhythmias with sotalol; propranolol fx also ↑d by chlorpromazine).

Dose: 25–300 mg tds po[BNF] (↓dose in elderly: 10 mg od may suffice); 25–50 mg tds/qds im (painful, and may ⇒ ↓BP/↑HR).

CICLOSPORIN

Calcineurin inhibitor: ⇒ ↓IL-2-mediated LØ proliferation.

Use: immunosuppression (esp post-transplant and in nephrotic syndrome).

CI (*only apply if given for nephrotic syndrome*): uncontrolled infection or HTN, malignancy.

Caution: HTN, ↑urate, porphyria, **L/R/P/B**.

SE: nephrotoxicity and **tremor** (both dose-related), ↑BP, hepatotoxicity, GI upset, biochemical Δs (↑K^+, ↑urate/gout, ↓Mg^{++}, ↑cholesterol). Rarely neuromuscular symptoms, HUS, Ca (esp lymphoma).

Warn: hypertrichosis, gingival hypertrophy, burning sensation in hands and feet.

Monitor: levels, LFTs, U&Es, Mg^{++}, lipids.

Interactions: metabolised by **P450**, ∴ many, particularly antibacterials and antifungals[BNF] (cephalosporins and penicillins

OK): levels esp ↓d by phenytoin and ↑d by erythromycin/clarithromycin and allopurinol.

Dose: specialist use[BNF]. Must prescribe by brand name (Neoral, Sandimmun or SangCya) as have different bioavailabilities and changing brands can ∴ ↓immunosuppression or ↑toxicity.

☠Check all new drugs for interactions before prescribing if on ciclosporin: ↑d levels ⇒ toxicity; ↓d levels may ⇒ rejection. ☠

CIMETIDINE
As ranitidine, but ↑↑interactions (↓**P450** & **W+**) and ↑gynaecomastia ∴ prescribed very rarely.

CIPROFLOXACIN
(Fluoro)quinolone antibiotic: inhibits DNA gyrase; 'cidal' with broad spectrum, but particularly good for Gram-negative infections.

Use: GI infections[1] (esp salmonella, shigella, campylobacter), **respiratory infections** (non-pneumococcal pneumonias[2], esp *Pseudomonas*). Also GU infections (esp UTIs[3], acute uncomplicated cystitis in women[4], gonorrhoea), 1st-line initial Rx of anthrax (*Bacillus anthracis*).

CI: quinolone allergy.

Caution: seizures (inc Hx of, or predisposition to), MG (can worsen), G6PD deficiency, children/adolescents (theoretical risk of arthropathy), R/P/B.

SE: GI upset (esp N&D, rarely AAC), **neuro-Ψ fx** (esp confusion, **seizures**; also headache, dizziness, hallucinations, sleep and mood Δs), **tendinitis ± rupture** (esp if elderly or taking steroids), **hypersensitivity**. Rarely hepatotoxicity, RF/interstitial nephritis, blood disorders, severe skin reactions (inc SJS, TEN).

Warn: avoid UV light*, avoid ingesting Fe- and Zn-containing products (e.g. antacids). May impair skilled tasks/driving.

Interactions: ↑s levels of theophyllines; NSAIDs ⇒ risk of seizures; ↑s nephrotoxicity of ciclosporin, FeSO$_4$ and antacids ⇒ ↓ciprofloxacin absorption (give 2 h before or 6 h after ciprofloxacin), **W+**.

Dose: 250–750 mg bd po, 100–400 mg bd ivi (each dose over 1 h) according to indication[BNF] (100 mg bd po for 3 days if cystitis).

☠ Stop if tendinitis, severe neuro-Ψ fx or hypersensitivity reaction. ☠

CITALOPRAM/CIPRAMIL
SSRI.
Use: depression[1] (and panic disorder). Useful if polypharmacy, as ↓interactions cf other SSRIs.
CI/Caution/SE: as fluoxetine.
Dose: 20 mg od[1] (↑ing if necessary to max 60 mg).

CITRAMAG see Bowel preparations
Dose: 1 sachet at 8am and 3pm the day before GI surgery or Ix.

CLARITHROMYCIN
Macrolide antibiotic: binds 50S ribosome; 'static' at low doses, 'cidal' at high doses.
Use: atypical pneumonias (as alternative to erythromycin; see p. 129), part of triple therapy for *H. pylori* (see p. 133).
CI/Caution/SE/Interactions: as erythromycin, but ⇒ ↓GI upset, **W+**.
Dose: 250–500 mg bd po or 500 mg bd iv.

CLEXANE see Enoxaparin

CLINDAMYCIN
Antibiotic; same action (but different structure and ∴ class) as clarithromycin; good against staphylococci (esp if resistant to penicillin) and anaerobes (esp bacteroides); penetrates bone well.
Use: osteomyelitis, intra-abdominal sepsis, endocarditis Px (limited dt SEs, esp AAC).
CI: diarrhoea.
Caution: L/R/P/B.

L/R/H = Liver, Renal and Heart failure (full key see p. x)

SE: GI upset (often ⇒ **AAC**), hepatotoxicity, blood disorders, local reactions at injection site, hypersensitivity.

Monitor: U&Es, LFTs.

Dose: 150–450 mg qds po; 0.6–4.8 g daily in divided doses im/ivi (doses >600 mg must be as ivi).

Stop drug if diarrhoea develops: AAC common and potentially fatal.

CLOBETASOL PROPIONATE CREAM (0.05%)/
DERMOVATE

Very-potent-strength topical corticosteroid.

CLOBETASONE BUTYRATE CREAM (0.05%)/
EUMOVATE

Moderately-potent-strength topical corticosteroid cream.

CLOMETHIAZOLE/HEMINEVRIN

Non-benzodiazepine hypnotic: no-hangover sedation, but high risk of dependence.

Use: alcohol withdrawal[1] (short-term Rx only), insomnia[2] (only in elderly).

CI: respiratory failure, alcoholics who continue to drink (⇒ risk of dependence, use only as part of inpatient detox regime).

Caution: Hx of drug abuse or respiratory/cardiac disease, L/R/E.

SE: headache, nasal/conjunctival irritation. Rarely paradoxical excitement, confusion, dependence, GI upset, rash, ΔLFTs, anaphylaxis.

Dose: 1–2 capsules nocte[2] (for alcohol withdrawal, see BNF).

CLOPIDOGREL/PLAVIX

Antiplatelet agent: ADP receptor antagonist. ↑antiplatelet fx cf aspirin (but also ↑SEs).

Use: Px of atherosclerotic events if Hx of ischaemic CVA, PVD or MI (esp with aspirin if ACS without ST elevation or pre-PCI).

CI: active bleeding, L (if severe – otherwise caution), **B**.

Caution: recent trauma, surgery, MI (for 1st few days after) or ischaemic CVA (for 1st week after), **R/P**.

SE: haemorrhage (esp GI or intracranial), GI upset, PU, headache, fatigue, dizziness, paraesthesia, rash/pruritus, hepatobiliary/blood disorders.

Dose: 75 mg od. If not already on clopidogrel, usually load with 300 mg for ACS then 75 mg od starting next day. If pre-PCI, load with 300 mg usually on morning of procedure.

Stop 7 days before operations if antiplatelet fx not wanted (e.g. major surgery); discuss with surgeons doing operation.

CLOTRIMAZOLE/CANESTEN

Imidazole antifungal (topical).
Use: external candida infections (esp vaginal thrush).
Caution: can damage condoms and diaphragms.
Dose: 2–3 applications/day of 1% cream, continuing for 14 days after lesion healed. Also available as powder/solution/spray for hairy areas, as pessary, and in 2% strength.

CLOZAPINE/CLOZARIL

Atypical antipsychotic: blocks dopamine ($D_4 > D_1 > D_{2\&3}$) and $5HT_{2A}$ receptors. Also mild blockade of muscarinic and adrenergic receptors.
Use: schizophrenia, but only if resistant or intolerant (e.g. severe extrapyramidal fx) to other antipsychotics[NICE].
CI: severe cardiac disorders (inc Hx of circulatory collapse, myocarditis, cardiomyopathy), coma/severe CNS depression, alcoholic/toxic psychosis, Hx of agranulocytosis or ↓NØ, bone marrow disorders, paralytic ileus, uncontrolled epilepsy, **R** (if severe, otherwise caution), **L/H/P/B**.
Caution: Hx of epilepsy, cardiovascular disease, ↑prostate, glaucoma (angle-closure), **E**.
SE: as olanzapine, but also can ⇒ ↓NØ (3% of patients) and ☠**agranulocytosis**☠ (1%). Also commonly ⇒ ↑salivation (Rx with hyoscine hydrobromide), ↓BP, constipation (can ⇒ ileus/obstruction:

have low threshold for giving laxatives), ↑Wt, sedation. Less
commonly seizures, urinary incontinence, myocarditis/ cardiomyopathy (*stop immediately!*), ↑HR, arrhythmias, hyperglycaemia,
N&V, ↑BP, delirium. Rarely hepatic dysfunction (*stop immediately!*),
↑TG, neuroleptic malignant syndrome.

Monitor: FBC*, serum levels and cardiac function (esp watch for
persistent ↑HR).

Interactions: as chlorpromazine, plus care with all drugs that
constipate, ↑QT threshold or ↓leukopoiesis (e.g. cytotoxics,
sulphonamides/cotrimoxazole, chloramphenicol, penicillamine,
carbamazepine, phenothiazines, esp depots). Caffeine, risperidone,
SSRIs (not citalopram), cimetidine and erythromycin ↑clozapine
levels. Smoking, carbamazepine and phenytoin ↓clozapine
levels.

Dose: initially 12.5 mg nocte, ↑ing to 200–450 mg /day[BNF] (max
900 mg/day).
If >2 days' doses missed, restart at 12.5 mg od and ↑gradually.

*Clozaril Patient Monitoring Service (tel: 0845 769 8269) can
provide practical advice about the drug, esp if blood disorder.
All patients must be registered before starting Rx for FBC and serum
level monitoring.

CO-AMILOFRUSE

Diuretic combination preparation for oedema that keeps K^+
stable: amiloride (K^+-sparing) + furosemide (K^+-wasting) in
3 strengths of tablet as 2.5/20, 5/40 and 10/80 (amiloride mg/
furosemide mg).

Dose: 1 tablet mane (NB: *specify strength!*).

CO-AMILOZIDE

Diuretic combination preparation for HTN, CCF and oedema.
Keeps K^+ stable: amiloride (K^+-sparing) + hydrochlorothiazide
(K^+-wasting) in 2 strengths of tablet as 2.5/25 and 5/50
(amiloride mg/hydrochlorothiazide mg).

Dose: ½–4 tablets daily, according to tablet strength and indication[BNF].

CO-AMOXICLAV

Combination of amoxicillin + clavulanic acid (β-lactamase inhibitor) to overcome resistance.

Use: UTIs, respiratory/skin/soft-tissue (plus many other) infections. Reserve for when β-lactamase-producing strains known/strongly suspected or other Rx has failed.

CI/Caution/SE: as ampicillin, plus **L** (↑risk of cholestasis), **P**.

Dose: 375 mg or 625 g tds po or 1.2 g tds iv (= combined dose of the 2 drugs). Non-proprietary and as Augmentin.

CO-BENELDOPA/MADOPAR

Combination of L-dopa and benserazide (peripheral dopa-decarboxylase inhibitor).

Use: parkinsonism.

CI/Caution/SE: see Levodopa.

Dose: (*expressed as levodopa only*) initially 50 mg tds/qds, ↑ing total dose and number of doses, according to response, to usual maintenance of 400–800 mg/day (↓ in elderly).

CO-CARELDOPA/SINEMET

Combination of L-dopa and carbidopa (peripheral dopa-decarboxylase inhibitor).

Use: parkinsonism.

CI/Caution/SE: see Levodopa.

Dose: (*expressed as levodopa only*) initially 50–100 mg tds, ↑ing total dose and number of doses, according to response, to usual maintenance of 400–800 mg/day (↓ in elderly).

CO-CODAMOL (8/500) = codeine 8 mg + paracetamol 500 mg per tablet.

Dose: 2 tablets qds prn.

CO-DANTHRAMER see Dantron; stimulant laxative.

Dose: 1–2 capsules or 5–10 ml suspension nocte (available in regular and strong formulations).

CO-DANTHRUSATE see Dantron; stimulant laxative.
Dose: 1–3 capsules or 5–15 ml suspension nocte.

CODEINE (PHOSPHATE)
Opioid analgesic.
Use: mild/moderate pain, diarrhoea, cough (as linctus).
CI/Caution/SE: as morphine, but milder SEs (**constipation** is the major problem: dose- and length of Rx-dependent; anticipate this and give laxative Px).
Dose: 30–60 mg up to qds po/im.

CO-DYDRAMOL = dihydrocodeine 10 mg + paracetamol
500 mg per tablet.
Dose: 2 tablets qds po prn.

COLCHICINE
Anti-gout: binds to tubulin of leukocytes and stops their migration to uric acid deposits ∴ ⇒ ↓inflammation. NB: slow action (needs >6 h to work).
Use: gout: acute attacks and as Px whilst waiting for allopurinol* (which may also initially worsen symptoms) and other drugs to work.
CI: P
Caution: GI diseases, L/H/R/B/E.
SE: GI upset (**N&V&D** and **abdominal pain** – all common and dose-related). Rarely GI haemorrhage, hypersensitivity, renal/hepatic impairment, peripheral neuritis, myopathy, alopecia, ↓spermatogenesis (reversible), blood disorders (if prolonged Rx).
Interactions: macrolides (esp erythromycin) ↑colchicine levels, loop diuretics ↓colchicine fx.
Dose: 0.5 mg tds for 7 days (start ASAP after symptom onset). More aggressive loading regimes exist[BNF] but ⇒ ↑GI upset w/o significant ↑ in response. Continue 0.5 mg tds for 3 months when starting allopurinol*.

CO-PROXAMOL = dextropropoxyphene* (mild opiate)
32.5 mg + paracetamol 325 mg per tablet.

Dose: 2 tablets qds po prn.

*Can $\Rightarrow$ HF in OD $\therefore$ less safe than other mild 'combination' analgesics.

CORSODYL Chlorhexidine mouthwash for Rx/Px of mouth infections (inc MRSA eradication); see local infection protocol.

CO-TRIAMTERZIDE

Diuretic combination preparation for HTN[1] and oedema[2]: triamterene (K^+-sparing) + hydrochlorothiazide (K^+-wasting) to keep K^+ stable.

Dose: initially 1 tablet[1] (or 2 tablets[2]) mane of 50/25 strength (= 50 mg triamterene + 25 mg hydrochlorothiazide), $\uparrow$ing if necessary to max of 4 tablets/day.

CO-TRIMOXAZOLE/SEPTRIN

Antibiotic combination preparation: 5 to 1 mixture of sulfamethoxazole (a sulphonamide) + trimethoprim $\Rightarrow$ synergistic action (individually are 'static' but collectively are 'cidal').

Use: PCP; other uses limited due to SEs (also rarely used for toxoplasmosis and nocardiasis).

CI: porphyria, **L** (if severe – otherwise only caution).

Caution: blood disorders, asthma, G6PD deficiency, **R/B/E**.

SE: skin reactions (inc SJS, TEN), **blood disorders** ($\downarrow$NØ, $\downarrow$Pt, BM suppression, agranulocytosis) relatively common, esp in elderly. Also N&V&D (inc AAC), nephrotoxicity, hepatotoxicity, hypersensitivity, anorexia, abdominal pain, glossitis, stomatitis, pancreatitis, arthralgia, myalgia, SLE, pulmonary infiltrates, seizures.

Interactions: $\uparrow$s fx of phenytoin and methotrexate (and, less so, sulphonylureas). $\downarrow$s fx of TCAs, **W+**.

Dose: PCP Rx: 120 mg/kg/day po/ivi in 2–4 divided doses (PCP Px 480–960 mg od po).

☠Stop immediately if rash or blood disorder occurs.☠

CYCLIZINE

Antihistamine antiemetic.

Use: N&V Rx/Px (esp 2° to iv/im opioids, but not 1st choice in angina/MI/LVF*), vertigo, motion sickness, labyrinthine disorders.

CI/Caution/SE: as chlorphenamine, but also avoid in severe HF* (may undo haemodynamic benefits of opioids). Antimuscarinic fx (see p. 174) are most prominent SEs.

Dose: 50 mg po/im/iv tds.

CYCLOPHOSPHAMIDE

Immunosuppressant, cytotoxic: alkylating agent (cross-links DNA bases, ↓ing replication).

Use: Ca, autoimmune diseases: esp vasculitis (inc rheumatoid arthritis, polymyositis and SLE (esp if renal/cerebral involvement)), systemic sclerosis, Wegener's, nephrotic syndrome in children.

CI: haemorrhagic cystitis.

Caution: BM suppression, L/R/P/B.

SE: GI upset, **alopecia** (reversible). Others rare but important: hepatotoxicity, blood disorders, malignancy (esp acute non-lymphocytic leukaemia), ↓**fertility** (can be permanent), pulmonary fibrosis (at high doses), **haemorrhagic cystitis** (only if given iv: ensure good hydration, give 'mesna' as Px; can occur months after Rx).

Warn: ↓fertility may be permanent (bank sperm if possible) – need to counsel and obtain consent regarding this before giving.

Dose: specialist use only.

☠ Stop immediately if rash or blood disorder occurs. ☠

CYCLOSPORIN see Ciclosporin

CYPROTERONE ACETATE

Anti-androgen.

Use: Ca prostate[1] (as adjunct), acne[2] (esp 2° to PCOS, where used with ethinylestradiol as co-cyprindiol), rarely for hypersexuality/ sexual deviation[3] (*males only!*).

CI: (*none apply if for Ca prostate*) advanced DM (if vascular disease), sickle cell, malignancy/wasting diseases, Hx of TE, age <18 years (can ⇒ ↓bone/testicular development), severe depression, **L/P**.
SE: fatigue, gynaecomastia, ↑ or ↓Wt, hepatotoxicity, blood disorders, hypersensitivity, osteoporosis, ↓spermatogenesis (reversible).
Monitor: FBC, LFTs, adrenocortical function.
Warn: driving and other skilled tasks may be impaired.
Dose: 200–300 mg po daily in divided doses[1], 50 mg bd po[3].

DALTEPARIN/FRAGMIN

Low-molecular-weight heparin (LMWH).
Use: DVT/PE Rx[1] and Px[2] (inc preoperative), MI/unstable angina[3].
CI/Caution/SE: see Heparin.
Dose: *all sc:* 200 units/kg (max 18 000 units) od[1]; 2500–5000 units od (according to risk[BNF])[2]; 120 units/kg bd for 8 days (max 10 000 units bd)[3]. Review dose after 8 days[BNF].

Monitoring (via anti Xa) needed if RF (i.e. creatinine >150), pregnancy, Wt >100 kg or <45 kg; see p. 158.

DANTRON

Stimulant laxative.
Use: constipation (use limited to terminally ill: theoretical risk of **carcinogenicity**).
Caution/SE: see Senna. (☠CI if GI obstruction☠)
Dose: see Co-danthramer and Co-danthrusate.

DERMOVATE see Clobetasol propionate cream 0.05%

DESFERRIOXAMINE

Fe (and Al) chelating agent.
Use: ↑Fe: acute (OD/poisoning[1]), chronic (e.g. xs transfusions for blood disorders, haemochromatosis when venesection CI). Also for ↑Al (e.g. 2° to dialysis).

L/R/H = Liver, Renal and Heart failure (full key see p. x)

Caution: Al-induced encephalopathy (may worsen), **R/P/B**.
SE: ↓**BP** (related to rate of ivi), lens opacities, retinopathy, GI upset,
blood disorders, hypersensitivity. Also neurological/respiratory/renal
dysfunction.
Monitor: vision and hearing during chronic Rx.
Dose: acutely up to 15 mg/kg/h ivi (max 80 mg/kg/day)[1]. Otherwise
according to degree of Fe or Al overload[BNF].

DEXAMETHASONE PHOSPHATE

Glucocorticoid; minimal mineralocorticoid activity, long duration
of action (see p. 169).
Use: cerebral oedema, Dx of Cushing's, N&V (2° to chemotherapy
or surgery), allergy/inflammation (esp if unresponsive shock),
congenital adrenal hyperplasia.
CI/Caution/SE: see Prednisolone and pp. 142–4.
Dose: cerebral oedema: acutely 10 mg iv, then 4 mg im qds (if not
life-threatening, some go straight to 4 mg qds iv then switch to
po a few days later). For other indications, see BNF/product
literature.

☠ Doses given here are for *dexamethasone phosphate* and must be
prescribed as such: other forms have different doses! ☠

DEXTROPROPOXYPHENE

Opioid (slightly milder than codeine), **W+**: used with paracetamol
as co-proxamol. *Unsafe in OD* (can ⇒ HF).

DF118 (suffix FORTE often omitted) Dihydrocodeine preparation.
Dose: 40–80 mg tds po with or after food (max 240 mg/day). 50 mg
sc/im 4–6 hourly.

NB: tablets are different dose to non-proprietary dihydrocodeine.

DIAMORPHINE

Strong opioid (1.5 × strength of morphine): analgesic, anxiolytic
and beneficial cardiac fx*: ↓s myocardial O_2 demand and
⇒ transient venodilation (↓s preload, cardiac filling pressures and
pulmonary congestion).

Use: severe pain[1]. Also acute MI[2], ACS[2] or LVF*[2].

CI/Caution/SE: see Morphine (but less ↓BP and nausea). **☠Respiratory depression** (esp elderly) and **constipation** ☠.

Dose: 5–10 mg sc/im (or ¼–½ this dose iv) up to 4-hourly[1]; 2.5–5 mg iv (at 1 mg/min)[2]. Can give as sc pump in chronic pain/palliative care; see pp. 142–4.

DIAZEMULS iv diazepam *emulsion*: ⇒ ↓venous irritation.

DIAZEPAM

Benzodiazepine, long-acting.

Use: seizures (esp status epilepticus[1], febrile convulsions), *short-term* Rx of acute alcohol withdrawal[2], anxiety[3], insomnia[4] (if also anxiety; if not, then shorter-acting forms preferred as ⇒ ↓hangover sedation). Also used for muscle spasm[5].

CI: respiratory depression/compromise (inc MG, sleep apnoea), chronic psychosis, depression (if diazepam alone given), phobic/obsessional states, **L** (if severe).

Caution: drug/alcohol abuse, personality disorder, porphyria, R/P/B/E.

SE: respiratory depression, drowsiness, dependence. Also ataxia, amnesia, headache, vertigo, GI upset, jaundice, ↓BP, ↓HR, visual/libido/urinary disturbances.

Dose: for status epilepticus[1] and alcohol withdrawal[2], see pp. 185 and 147, respectively; 2 mg tds po (↑ up to 30 mg/day)[3,5]; 5–15 mg nocte po[4]. ↓dose if elderly or LF. If chronic exposure to benzodiazepines, ↑doses may be needed; do not stop suddenly, as can ⇒ withdrawal; see p. 171 for details.

☠**Respiratory depression**: if ↑doses used (esp iv/im), monitor O_2 sats and have flumazenil and O_2 (± intubation equipment) at hand – see p. 196 for Mx. ☠

DICLOFENAC

Medium-strength NSAID.

Use: pain/inflammation, esp musculoskeletal; rheumatoid arthritis, osteoarthritis, acute gout, postoperative (esp orthopaedic).

CI/Caution/ SE: see Ibuprofen (risk of GI ulcer/bleeds can be ↓d by combination with misoprostol as Arthrotec).
Dose: 50 mg tds po or 75 mg bd po (or im, but for max of 2 days), 100 mg od pr (max 150 mg/day). Rarely used iv[BNF].

DIDRONEL PMO see Etidronate; bisphosphonate for osteoporosis.

DIFFLAM Benzydamine: topical NSAID.
Use: mouth ulcers, radio/chemotherapy-induced mucositis as spray (4–8 sprays 1.5–3-hourly) or oral rinse (15 ml 1.5–3-hourly). Available as cream for musculoskeletal pain.

DIGIBIND Anti-digoxin Ab for digoxin toxicity/OD unresponsive to supportive Rx. See product literature for dose.

DIGOXIN
Cardiac glycoside: ↓s HR by slowing AVN conduction and ↑ing vagal tone. Also weak inotrope.
Use: AF (and other SVTs), HF.
CI: HB (intermittent complete), 2nd-degree AV block, HOCM (can use with care if also AF and HF), SVTs 2° to WPW.
Caution: recent MI, ↓K⁺*/↓T₄ (both ⇒ ↑digoxin toxicity*), SSS. R/P/E.
SE: generally mild unless rapid ivi, xs Rx or OD: **GI upset** (esp nausea), **arrhythmias/HB, neuro-Ψ disturbances** (inc visual Δs, esp blurred vision and yellow/green halos), fatigue, weakness, confusion, hallucinations, mood Δs. Also gynaecomastia (if chronic Rx), rarely ↓Pt, rash.
Monitor: U&Es, digoxin levels (ideally take 6 h post-dose: therapeutic range 1–2 μg/l).
Interactions: digoxin fx/toxicity ↑d by Ca⁺⁺ antagonists (esp verapamil), amiodarone, propafenone, quinidine, antimalarials, itraconazole, amphotericin, ciclosporin, diuretics (mostly via ↓K⁺*), but also ACE-i/AII antagonists and spironolactone despite potential ↑K⁺. Cholestyramine and antacids can ↓ digoxin absorption.

Dose: *non-acute:* load with 125–250 µg bd po (maintenance dose 62.5–375 µg od). ↓dose if RF or elderly.

Digoxin loading for acute AF: *either* 0.75–1 mg as ivi over 2 h *or* 500 µg po repeated 12 h later. Then follow non-acute schedule.

DIHYDROCODEINE see Codeine; similar-strength opioid analgesic.
Dose: 30–60 mg up to qds po (or up to 50 mg qds im/sc) with or after food. ↑doses can be given under close supervision.

DILATING EYE DROPS for fundoscopy:
1 **Tropicamide 1%** Most common; avoid if Hx of angle-closure glaucoma (cloudy cornea should raise suspicion) but OK if open-angle/simple glaucoma.
2 **Phenylephrine 2.5% or 10%** Better for Asian and black patients, as ↓ response to tropicamide is common. CI if angle closure glaucoma and avoid if limbal ischaemia (e.g. after chemical injury).
Consider cycloplegic forms (e.g. cyclopentolate) for children or if corneal abrasions, as they are more comfortable for examination.

DILTIAZEM
Rate-limiting benzothiazepine Ca^{++} channel blocker: ↓s HR and contractility* (but <verapamil) and ↓s BP. Also dilates peripheral/coronary arteries.
Use: Rx/Px of angina[1] (esp if β-blockers CI) and HTN[2].
CI: LVF* (can worsen), ↓↓HR, 2nd/3rd-degree HB, SSS, **P/B**.
Caution: 1st-degree HB, ↑PR interval, **L/R/H**.
SE: headache, flushing, GI upset (esp **N&C**), **oedema** (esp ankle), ↓HR, ↓BP. Rarely SAN/AVN block, arrhythmias, rash, hepatotoxicity.
Interactions: β-blockers and verapamil (can ⇒ asystole, AV block, ↓↓HR, HF). ↑s fx of digoxin, ciclosporin, theophyllines, carbamazepine and phenytoin.
Dose: 60 mg tds (↑ing to max of 360 mg/day)[1]; 180–480 mg/day in 1 or 2 doses[2] (*suitable for HTN only as MR preparation: no*

non-proprietary forms exist and brands vary in clinical fx ∴ specify which is required[BNF]). Consider ↓ing doses if LF or RF.

DIPROBASE Paraffin-based emollient cream/ointment for dry skin conditions (e.g. eczema, psoriasis).

DIPYRIDAMOLE/PERSANTIN
Antiplatelet agent: inhibits Pt aggregation (also ⟹ arterial dilation: inc coronaries).
Use: 2° prevention of ischaemic TIA/CVA[1], Px of TE from prosthetic valves (as adjunct to warfarin)[2].
Caution: recent MI, angina (if unstable), aortic stenosis, ↓BP, MG*, migraine (may worsen), **H**.
SE: GI upset, dizziness, myalgia, headache, ↓BP, ↑HR, hot flushes, rarely worsening of IHD, hypersensitivity (rash, urticaria, bronchospasm, angioedema), ↑postoperative bleeding, ↓Pt.
Interactions: ↓s fx of cholinesterase inhibitors*, ↑s fx of adenosine. Fx of dipyridamole ↓d by theophyllines, **W+**.
Dose: 200 mg bd as MR preparation (Persantin retard)[1]; 100–200 mg tds[2]. All doses to be taken with food.

DISULFIRAM/ANTABUSE
Alcohol dehydrogenase inhibitor: ⟹ ↑systemic acetaldehyde ⟹ unpleasant SE when alcohol ingested (inc small amounts ∴ care with alcohol-containing medications, foods, toiletries).
Use: alcohol withdrawal (maintenance of).
CI: Hx of IHD or CVA, HTN, psychosis, ↑suicide risk, severe personality disorder, **H/P/B**.
Caution: DM, epilepsy, respiratory disease, **L/R**.
SE: only if alcohol ingested – N&V, flushing, headache, ↑HR, ↓BP (± collapse if xs alcohol intake).
Interactions: ↑s fx of phenytoin, **W+**.
Dose: initially 800 mg od, ↓ing to 100–200 mg od over 5 days.
NB: Must have consumed no alcohol within at least 24 h of 1st dose.

DOBUTAMINE

Inotropic sympathomimetic: mostly β_1 fx $\Rightarrow$ ↑contractility. ↓fx on HR cf dopamine.

Use: shock (cardiogenic, septic).

Caution: severe ↓BP.

SE: ↑HR, ↑BP (if xs Rx).

Dose: 2.5–10 μg/kg/min ivi, titrating to response (via central line, preferably with invasive cardiac monitoring). Often given with dopamine; seek expert help.

DOCUSATE SODIUM

Stimulant laxative: $\Rightarrow$ ↑GI motility (also a softening agent).

Use/Caution/SE: see Senna (☠ **CI if GI obstruction** ☠).

Dose: 50–100 mg up to tds po (max 500 mg/day). Also available as enemas[BNF].

DOMPERIDONE

Antiemetic: D_2 antagonist – inhibits central nausea chemoreceptor trigger zone. Poor BBB penetration ∴ ↓central SEs (extrapyramidal fx, sedation) cf other dopamine antagonists.

Use: N&V, esp 2° to chemotherapy and morning-after pill, and in Parkinson's disease.

Caution: GI obstruction **P/B**.

SE: rash, allergy, ↑prolactin (can $\Rightarrow$ gynaecomastia and galactorrhoea). Rarely ↓libido, dystonia.

Dose: 10 mg tds po (can ↑ to max 20 mg 4-hourly) or 30 mg tds pr (can ↑ to 60 mg 4-hourly). Not available im/iv.

DONEPEZIL/ARICEPT

Acetylcholinesterase inhibitor.

Use: Alzheimer's disease[NICE].

CI: P/B.

Caution: supraventricular conduction dfx (esp SSS), ↑risk of PU (e.g. Hx of PU or NSAID), COPD/asthma, extrapyramidal symptoms can worsen, **L**.

L/R/H = Liver, Renal and Heart failure (full key see p. x)

SE: cholinergic fx (see p. 174), **GI upset, insomnia, headache,**
fatigue, dizziness, syncope, rash, Ψ disturbances. Rarely $\downarrow$ or $\uparrow$BP,
seizures, PU/GI bleeds, SAN/AVN block, hepatotoxicity.
Dose: 5 mg nocte ($\uparrow$ to 10 mg after 1 month if necessary); specialist
use only – need review for clinical response and tolerance.

DOPAMINE

Inotropic sympathomimetic: dose-dependent fx on receptors: low
doses (2–3 µg/kg/min) stimulate peripheral DA receptors but little
else $\therefore \Rightarrow \uparrow$renal perfusion*; higher doses (>5 µg/kg/min) also have
β_1 fx ($\Rightarrow \uparrow$ contractility), even higher doses have α fx ($\Rightarrow$ vasoconstriction, but can worsen HF).
Use: shock, esp if ARF* or cardiogenic (e.g. post-MI or cardiac
surgery).
CI: tachyarrhythmias, phaeo.
SE: N&V, $\downarrow$ or $\uparrow$BP, $\uparrow$HR, peripheral vasoconstriction.
Dose: initially 2–5 µg/kg/min ivi (via central line, preferably with
invasive cardiac monitoring), then adjust to response; seek specialist
help.

DORZOLAMIDE/TRUSOPT

Topical carbonic anhydrase inhibitor: see Acetazolamide (oral
preparation; more potent drug but with more SEs).
Use: glaucoma (esp if β-blocker CI or fails to $\downarrow$IOP).
CI: $\uparrow$Cl$^-$ acidosis, **R** (severe only), **P/B**.
Caution: Hx of renal stones* or intraocular surgery, corneal dfx, **L**.
SE: local irritation, blurred vision, bitter taste, anterior uveitis, rash &
urolithiasis*. Some systemic SEs occur (much less than oral/iv preps:
see acetazolamide).
Dose: apply 2% drop tds. Also available in bd preps with timolol
(Cosopt).

DOXAPRAM

Respiratory stimulant: $\uparrow$s activity of respiratory and vasomotor centres
in medulla $\Rightarrow \uparrow$depth (and, to lesser extent, rate) of breathing. Also
indirect fx by stimulation of chemoreceptors in aorta and carotid artery.

Use: hypoventilation, life-threatening respiratory failure – usually only if dt transient/reversible cause, e.g. postoperative/post-general anaesthetic, acute deterioration w known precipitant. Mostly used in preventing respiratory depression $2°$ to $\uparrow FiO_2$ used in severe respiratory acidosis (can be harmful if $CO_2 \downarrow$ or normal).
CI: severe asthma or HTN, IHD, $\uparrow T_4$, epilepsy, physical obstruction of respiratory tract.
Caution: if taking MAOIs, L/H/P.
SE: headache, flushing, chest pains, arrhythmias, vasoconstriction, $\uparrow BP$, $\uparrow HR$, laryngo/bronchospasm, GI upset, dizziness, seizures.
Dose: specialist use only (mostly in ITU).

DOXAZOSIN/CARDURA

α_1 blocker $\Rightarrow$ systemic vasodilation and relaxation of internal urethral sphincter $\therefore \Rightarrow \downarrow TPR^1$ and $\uparrow$bladder outflow[2].
Use: HTN[1], BPH[2].
CI: postural $\downarrow BP$, micturition syncope.
Caution: L/R/H/P/B/E.
SE: postural $\downarrow BP$ (esp after 1st dose*), **dizziness**, **headache**, **urinary incontinence** (esp women), GI upset (esp N&V), drowsiness/fatigue, syncope, mood Δs, dry mouth, oedema, somnolence, blurred vision, rhinitis. Rarely erectile dysfunction, $\uparrow HR$, arrhythmias, hypersensitivity/rash. Chronic Rx $\Rightarrow$ beneficial lipid Δs ($\uparrow HDL$, $\downarrow LDL$, $\downarrow VLDL$, $\downarrow TG$).
Interactions: $\uparrow$s hypotensive fx of diuretics, β-blockers, Ca^{++} antagonists and antidepressants.
Dose: initially 1 mg od (give 1st dose before bed*), then slowly $\uparrow$ according to response (max 16 mg/day[1] or 8 mg/day[2]). 4 or 8 mg od if MR preparation, as Cardura XL.

DOXYCYCLINE

Tetracycline antibiotic: inhibits ribosomal (30S) subunit. Has longest $t_{1/2}$ of all tetracyclines $\therefore$ od dosing.
Use: **genital infections**, esp syphilis, chlamydia, PID, salpingitis, urethritis (non-gonococcal). Also **tropical diseases**, e.g. rickettsia (inc Q fever), *Brucella*, Lyme disease (*Borrelia*

burgdorferi), malaria (Px/Rx, not 1st-line), mycoplasma (respiratory/genital), COPD infective exac (*H. influenzae*), **anthrax** (Rx/Px).
CI/Caution/SE: as tetracycline, but can give with caution if RF.
Warn: avoid UV light; avoid taking Zn- and Fe-containing products (e.g. antacids).
Dose: 100–200 mg od/bd[BNF].

EDROPHONIUM
Short-acting anticholinesterase given iv/im during Tensilon test for Dx of MG – look for ↓symptoms (i.e. ↑strength).

ENALAPRIL/INNOVACE
ACE-i.
Use/CI/Caution/SE: see Captopril.
Dose: initially 2.5 mg od (5 mg if for HTN and not elderly, on diuretics or RF), then ↑ according to response (max 40 mg od).

ENOXAPARIN/CLEXANE
Low-molecular-weight heparin (LMWH).
Use: DVT/PE Rx[1] and Px[2] (inc preoperative), MI/unstable angina Rx/Px[3].
CI/Caution/SE: see Heparin.
Dose: (all sc; 1 mg = 100 units) 1.5 mg/kg od[1], 40 mg od (20 mg od if not high risk)[2], 1 mg/kg bd[3].
Monitoring (via anti Xa) needed if RF (i.e. creatinine >150), pregnancy, Wt >100 kg or <45 kg; see p. 158.

ENSURE Protein- and calorie-rich drinks for undernourished patients.

EPILIM see Valproate

EPINEPHRINE see Adrenaline

EPOETIN

Recombinant erythropoietin.

Use: ↓Hb 2° to CRF (and rarely 2° to AZT or platinum-containing chemotherapy). 3 types: α (Eprex), β (NeoRecormon) and longer-acting darbepoetin (▼Aranesp).

SE: ↑BP, ↑K+, seizures. ☠ Eprex **rarely ⇒ red cell aplasia (esp in sc form which is now contraindicated).** ☠

Dose: sc (self-administered), iv (inpatients)[BNF]. Check Fe levels are replete before starting.

EPROSARTAN/TEVETEN

Angiotensin II antagonist.

Use: HTN

CI: L (if severe), **P**.

Caution/SE/Interactions: see Losartan.

Dose: 600 mg od (max 800 mg od). Start at 300 mg and then ↑ as required if elderly, RF or LF.

EPTIFIBATIDE/INTEGRILIN

Antiplatelet agent: glycoprotein IIb/IIIa receptor inhibitor ∴ stops binding of fibrinogen and inhibits Pt aggregation.

Use: Px of MI in unstable angina and NSTEMI (if last episode of chest pain <24 h ago), esp if high risk and awaiting PCI[NICE] (see p. 180).

CI: active or ↑risk of bleeding; bleeding disorder, severe trauma or major surgery w/in 6 weeks, abnormal bleeding or CVA w/in 30 days, Hx of haemorrhagic CVA or intracranial disease (AVM, aneurysm or neoplasm), ↓Pt ,↑INR, severe HTN, **L/R** (if either severe – otherwise caution), **B**.

Caution: drugs that ↑bleeding risk (esp thrombolysis), **P**.

SE: bleeding.

Monitor: FBC 6 h after starting and daily thereafter.

Dose: initially 180 µg/kg iv bolus followed by ivi of 2 µg/kg/min for up to 72 h (or 96 h if awaiting PCI). Needs concurrent heparin: LMWH is simplest, and patients are usually already on this.

Specialist use only: get senior advice or contact on-call cardiology.

L/R/H = Liver, Renal and Heart failure (full key see p. x)

ERGOCALCIFEROL (= CALCIFEROL)

Vitamin D_2: requires renal (1) and hepatic (25) hydroxylation for activation.

Use: vitamin D deficiency.

CI: $\uparrow Ca^{++}$, metastatic calcification.

Caution: R (B if high 'pharmacological'* doses used).

SE: $\uparrow Ca^{++}$. If over-Rx: **GI upset**, weakness, headache, polydipsia/polyuria, anorexia, RF, arrhythmias.

Monitor: Ca^{++} (esp if N&V develops).

Dose: 10–20 µg od as part of multivitamin preparations or combined with calcium lactate or phosphate as 'calcium + ergocalciferol': non-proprietary preparations are available but it is often prescribed by trade name (e.g. Cacit D3, or Calcichew D3). $\uparrow$doses of 0.25–1.0 mg od (of 'pharma-cological strength' preparations*) used for GI malabsorption and chronic liver disease causes (up to 2.5 mg od for hypoparathyroidism).

*Specify strength of tablet required to avoid confusion[BNF].

ERYTHROMYCIN

Macrolide antibiotic: binds 50S ribosome; 'static' at low doses, 'cidal' at high doses.

Use: atypical pneumonias (with other agents; see p. 129), rarely *Chlamydia*/other GU infections, *Campylobacter enteritis*. Often used if allergy to penicillin.

Caution: $\uparrow$QTc, porphyria, L/R/P/B.

SE: GI upset (rarely AAC), **dry itchy skin**, hypersensitivity (inc SJS, TEN), arrhythmias (esp VT), chest pain, reversible hearing loss (dose-related, esp if RF), cholestatic jaundice.

Interactions: $\downarrow$P450 $\therefore$ many; most importantly $\uparrow$s levels of ciclosporin, digoxin, theophyllines and carbamazepine, **W+**.

Dose: 500 mg qds po (250 mg qds if mild infection, 1 g qds if severe); 50 mg/kg daily iv in 4 divided doses (NB: venous irritant $\therefore$ give po if possible).

ESMOLOL

β-blocker: cardioselective ($\beta_1 > \beta_2$) and short-acting*.
Use: SVTs (inc AF, atrial flutter, sinus ↑HR), HTN (esp
perioperatively), acute MI (*safer than long-acting preparations).
CI/Caution/SE: see Propranolol.
Dose: usually 50–200 µg/kg/min ivi, preceded by loading dose if
perioperative (see product literature). Also see NCT algorithm in
inside front cover.

▼ETANERCEPT/ENBREL

Monoclonal Ab against TNF-α (an inflammatory cytokine).
Use: Crohn's disease and rheumatoid/psoriatic arthritis resistant to
standard DMARDs (steroids or other immunosuppression)^NICE. Also
juvenile idiopathic arthritis.
CI/Caution: See product literature.
SE: blood disorders, severe infections, CNS demyelination, GI
upset, exac of HF, headache. *Specialist use only.*
☠ Do not give live vaccines during Rx. ☠

ETHAMBUTOL

Anti-TB antibiotic: inhibits cell-wall synthesis ('static').
Use: TB initial Rx phase (1st 2 months) *if isoniazid resistance
known or suspected* (see p. 131).
CI: optic neuritis, ↓vision.
Caution: **R** (monitor levels* and ↓dose if creatinine clearance
<30 ml/min), **P/E**.
SE: neuritis; peripheral and **optic** (can ⇒ ↓visual acuity**,
colour-blindness, ↓visual fields ∴ ⇒ baseline and regular
ophthalmology review). Rarely GI upset, skin reactions, ↓Pt.
Warn: patient to report immediately any visual symptoms – use
alternative drug if unable to do this (e.g. very young, ↓IQ).
Monitor: visual acuity** (inc baseline before Rx), plasma levels*.
Dose: 15 mg/kg od (30 mg/kg 3 times a week if 'supervised' Rx).

(DISODIUM) ETIDRONATE

Bisphosphonate: ↓s bone turnover.

Use: osteoporosis Rx/Px[1] (if alendronate or risedronate not suitable/tolerated), Paget's disease[2].
CI: R (only caution if mild – ↓dose), **P/B**.
SE: GI upset, ↑PO_4 (transient *NB: other bisphosphonates* ↓PO_4!).
Can ⇒ bone pain in Paget's disease (stop if ⇒ fractures). Rarely, neurological disorders (headache, paraesthesia, peripheral neuropathy), blood disorders, hypersensitivity/skin reactions.
Monitor: ALP, Ca^{++}, PO_4 (and urinary hydroxyproline[2]).
Warn: avoid food for ≥2 h after taking, esp Ca^{++}-containing products (milk, Fe/mineral supplements, antacids).
Dose: 400 mg for 14 days followed by 1.25 g $CaCO_3$ for 76 days (as Didronel PMO in 90-day packs: 1 tablet od)[1]; 5–20 mg/kg od pp[2].

ETODOLAC
Medium-strength NSAID, selective COX2 inhibitor.
Use: osteo- or rheumatoid arthritis symptom relief[NICE].
CI/Caution/SE: see Celecoxib.
Dose: 300 mg bd (or 600 mg od as Lodine SR).

▼ETORICOXIB/ARCOXIA
NSAID, selective COX2 inhibitor.
Use: osteo-/rheumatoid arthritis, other pain (musculoskeletal, dental, acute gout, dysmenorrhoea)[NICE].
CI/Caution/SE: see Celecoxib.
Dose: 60–120 mg od.

EUMOVATE see Clobetasone butyrate 0.05%; moderate-strength steroid cream.

FANSIDAR
Antimalarial: combination tablet of pyrimethamine (25 mg) + sulfadoxine (500 mg).
Use: Rx of falciparum malaria (with or following quinine).
CI: sulphonamide allergy, porphyria.
Caution: blood disorders, asthma, G6PD deficiency, **L/R/P/B/E**.
SE: blood disorders, **skin reactions**, pulmonary infiltrates, insomnia, GI upset, nephrotoxicity, hepatotoxicity, hypersensitivity.

Monitor: FBC if chronic Rx.
Dose: see p. 134.

FENTANYL/DUROGESIC

Strong opiate used mostly as topical slow-release patch in chronic, severe, intractable pain.
CI/Caution/SE: see Morphine.
Dose: four patch strengths: 25, 50, 75 and 100, which denote release of μg/h (to calculate initial dose, these are equivalent to daily oral morphine requirement of 90, 180, 270 and 360 mg, respectively). Replace every 72 h.
NB ↑fx and SEs if fever or external heat (↑absorption can occur).

FERROUS SULPHATE

Oral Fe preparation.
Use: Fe-deficient ↓Hb Rx/Px.
Caution: P.
SE: dark stools (can confuse with melaena, which smells worse!), GI upset (take with food if problematic, but ⇒ ↓absorption), Δ bowel habit (dose-dependent).
Dose: 200 mg tds (od/bd for Px).

FINASTERIDE

Antiandrogen: 5-α-reductase inhibitor: ↓s testosterone conversion to more potent dihydrotestosterone.
Use: BPH[1] (⇒ ↓prostate size and ∴ symptomatic relief), male-pattern baldness[2].
Caution: Ca prostate (can ⇒ ↓PSA & ∴ mask), obstructive uropathy, P (teratogenic; although not taken by women, partners of those on the drug can absorb it from crushed tablets and semen, in which it is excreted ∴ *females must avoid handling tablets, and sexual partners of those on the drug must use condoms if, or likely to become, pregnant*).
SE: sexual dysfunction, testicular pain, gynaecomastia, hypersensitivity (inc swelling of lips/face).
Dose: 5 mg od[1] (Proscar), 1 mg od[2] (▼Propecia).

FLAGYL see Metronidazole

FLECAINIDE
Class Ic antiarrhythmic; local anaesthetic.
Use: VT[1] (if serious and symptomatic), SVT[2] (esp junctional re-entry tachycardias and paroxysmal AF).
CI: chronic AF (with no attempts at cardioversion), Hx of MI and asymptomatic VEs or non-sustained VT, valvular heart disease (if haemodynamically compromised), **H.**
Caution: pacemakers, SAN dysfunction, atrial conduction dfx, AF post cardiac surgery, HB (not 1st-degree), BBB, L/R/P/B/E.
SE: GI upset, syncope, dyspnoea, vision/mood disturbances. Rarely **arrhythmias**.
Monitor: plasma levels in RF (keep at 0.2–1 mg/l), ECG if giving iv.
Interactions: levels ↑d by amiodarone, fluoxetine and quinine. ↑s digoxin levels. Myocardial depression may occur with β-blockers/verapamil.
Dose: initially 100 mg bd po, ↓ing after 3–5 days if possible (max 400 mg/day)[1]; 50 mg bd po, ↑ing if necessary to 300 mg/day[2]. Acutely, 2 mg/kg iv over 10–30 min (max 150 mg), then (if required) 1.5 mg/kg/h ivi for 1 h, then ↓ing to 100–250 µg/kg/h for up to 24 h, then give po (max cumulative dose in 1st 24 h = 600 mg).

FLEET (PHOSPHO-SODA) see Bowel preparations
Dose: 45 ml (mixed with 120 ml water, then followed by 240 ml water) taken twice: for morning procedures, at 7am and 7pm the day before; for afternoon procedures, at 7pm the day before and at 7am on the day of procedure.

FLIXOTIDE see Fluticasone (inh steroid). 50, 100, 250 or 500 µg/puff as powder. 25, 50, 125 or 250 µg/puff as aerosol.
Dose: 100–2000 µg/day (aerosol doses <powder doses).

FLOMAX see Tamsulosin

FLUCLOXACILLIN

Penicillin (penicillinase-resistant).

Use: penicillin-resistant (β-lactamase-producing) staphylococcal infections, esp skin[1] (surgical wounds, Venflon sites, cellulitis, impetigo, otitis externa), rarely as adjunct in pneumonia[1]. Also osteomyelitis[2], endocarditis[3].

CI/Caution/SE: as benzylpenicillin, plus rarely hepatitis, **cholestatic jaundice** (may develop after Rx stopped).

Dose: 250–500 mg qds po/im (or up to 2 g qds iv)[1]; up to 2 g qds iv[2]; 2 g 4-hourly iv for 4 wks[3].

FLUCONAZOLE

Triazole antifungal: good po absorption and CSF penetration.

Use: fungal meningitis (esp cryptococcal), candidiasis (mucosal, vaginal, systemic), other fungal infections (esp tinea, pittyria).

Caution: L/R/P/B.

SE: GI upset, **hypersensitivity** (can ⇒ angioedema, TEN, SJS, anaphylaxis: if develops rash, stop drug or monitor closely), **hepatotoxicity**, headache. Rarely blood/metabolic ($\uparrow$lipids, $\downarrow K^+$) disorders, dizziness, seizures, alopecia.

Monitor: LFTs: stop drug if clinical features of liver disease develop.

Interactions: $\downarrow$**P450** ∴ many; most importantly, $\uparrow$s fx of theophyllines, ciclosporin and tacrolimus, **W+**.

Dose: 50–400 mg/day po/iv according to indication[BNF].

FLUDROCORTISONE

Mineralocorticoid.

Use: adrenocortical deficiency, esp Addison's disease[1].

SE: H_2O/Na^+ **retention**, $\downarrow K^+$ (monitor U&Es).

Dose: 50–300 µg/day po[1].

FLUMAZENIL

Benzodiazepine antagonist.

Use: benzodiazepine OD/toxicity (esp if respiratory depression).

CI: life-threatening conditions controlled by benzodiazepines (e.g. ↑ICP, status epilepticus).

Caution: mixed ODs (esp TCAs), benzodiazepine dependence (may ⇒ withdrawal fx; see p. 173), Hx of panic disorder (can ⇒ relapse), head injury, epileptics on long-term benzodiazepine Rx (may ⇒ fits), **L/P/B/E.**

SE: N&V, dizziness, blurred vision, headache, flushing, rebound anxiety/agitation, transient ↑BP/HR.

Dose: initially 0.2 mg over 30 s, then wait 30 s for response. If unsuccessful give 2nd dose of 0.3 mg, then subsequent doses of 0.5 mg. *Max total dose 3 mg.*

NB: short $t_{1/2}$ – observe closely after Rx and consider further doses.

☠Flumazenil is not recommended as a diagnostic test and should not be given routinely in overdoses as risk of inducing:

1 **fits** (esp if epileptic)
2 **withdrawal syndrome** (if habituated to benzodiazepines)
3 **arrhythmias** (esp if co-ingested TCA or amphetamine-like drug of abuse).
  If in any doubt get senior opinion and exclude habituation to benzodiazepines and get ECG before giving. ☠

!!

FLUOXETINE/PROZAC

SSRI: long $t_{1/2}$.

Use: depression, other Ψ disorders (inc bulimia, OCD).

CI: active mania.

Caution: epilepsy, receiving ECT, mania Hx, heart disease, DM*, glaucoma (angle-closure), ↑risk of bleeding, **L/R/H/P/B.**

Class SEs: GI upset, ↓Wt, **insomnia, agitation, headache, hypersensitivity, withdrawal fx** (headache, nausea, paraesthesia, dizziness, anxiety ∴ *stop slowly!*). Rarely extrapyramidal/ antimuscarinic fx (see p. 174), sexual dysfunction, convulsions, ↓Na⁺ (inc SIADH), blood disorders.

Specific SEs: rarely **hypoglycaemia*, vasculitis** (**rash** may be 1st sign).

Interactions: ↓**P450** ∴ many, but most importantly ↑s levels of TCAs, benzodiazepines, clozapine and haloperidol. ↑s lithium toxicity and ⇒ HTN and ↑CNS fx with selegiline (and other dopaminergics). Antagonises antiepileptics (but ↑s levels of carbamazepine and phenytoin). ☠*Never give with MAOIs.*☠ (Mild **W+**.)
Dose: 20 mg mane (max 60 mg).

FLUTICASONE/FLIXOTIDE (various delivery devices available[BNF])
Inhaled corticosteroid for asthma: see Beclometasone.
Dose: 100–2000 µg/day inh (or 0.5–2 mg bd as nebs).
1 µg equivalent to 2 µg of beclometasone or budesonide.

FOLIC ACID (= FOLATE)
Vitamin: building block of nucleic acids.
Use: megaloblastic ↓Hb Rx/Px if haemolysis/dialysis[1] (or GI malabsorption where ↑doses may be needed), Px against neural-tube dfx in pregnancy[2] (esp if on antiepileptics), Px of mucositis and GI upset if on methotrexate[3].
Caution: undiagnosed megaloblastic ↓Hb (i.e. ↓B_{12} not excluded) – *folate given without B_{12} in B_{12} deficiency can precipitate subacute combined degeneration of spinal cord.*
SE: malaise, bronchospasm, allergy.
Dose: 5 mg od[1] (in maintenance, ↓frequency of dose, often to weekly); 400 µg od[2] (unless mother has neural-tube defect herself or has previously had a child with a neural-tube defect, when 5 mg od needed); 5 mg once weekly[3].

FORMOTEROL (= EFORMOTEROL)/FORADIL, OXIS
Long-acting β_2 agonist 'LABA'; as Salmeterol plus **L**.
Dose: 6–36 µg od/bd inh (min and max doses vary between preparations[BNF]).

FOSPHENYTOIN
Antiepileptic: (new, expensive) prodrug of phenytoin – allows safer rapid loading.

Use: epilepsy (esp status epilepticus).
CI/Caution/SE: as phenytoin, but ↓SEs (esp ↓arrhythmias and 'purple glove syndrome').
Dose: see phenytoin (prescribe as 'phenytoin sodium equivalent'.
NB: fosphenytoin 1.5 mg = phenytoin 1 mg).

FRAGMIN see Dalteparin; low-molecular-weight heparin.

FRUMIL see Co-amilofruse; tablets are 5/40 (5 mg amilozide + 40 mg furosemide) unless stated as LS (= 2.5/20) or FORTE (= 10/80).

FRUSEMIDE now called furosemide

FUSIDIC ACID/FUCIDIN
Antibiotic; good bone penetration & activity against *S. aureus*.
Use: osteomyelitis, endocarditis (2° to penicillin-resistant staphylococci) – needs 2nd antibiotic to prevent resistance.
Caution: biliary disease or obstruction (⇒ ↓elimination), L/P/B.
SE: GI upset, hepatitis*. Rarely: skin reactions, blood disorders, ARF.
Monitor: LFTs*.
Dose: 500 mg tds po (↑ to 1 g tds in severe infections or 750 mg tds if using suspension); 500 mg tds iv (6–7 mg/kg tds if weight <50 kg).

FUROSEMIDE (previously FRUSEMIDE)
Loop diuretic: inhibits Na^+/K^+ pump in ascending loop of Henle ⇒ ↓resorption and ∴ ↑loss of $Na^+/K^+/Cl^-/H_2O$.
Use: LVF[1] (esp in acute pulmonary oedema, but also in chronic LVF/CCF or as Px during blood transfusion), HTN, oliguria secondary to ARF (after correcting hypovolaemia first).
CI: cirrhosis (if precomatose), **R** (if anuria).
Caution: ↓BP, ↑prostate, porphyria, L/P/B.
SE: ↓BP (inc postural), ↓K^+, ↓Na^+, ↓Ca^{++}, ↓Mg^{++}, ↓Cl^- alkalosis. Also ↑urate/gout, GI upset, ↑glucose/impaired glucose

tolerance, ↑cholesterol/TGs (temporary). Rarely **BM suppression**
(stop drug), RF, skin reactions, pancreatitis, tinnitus/deafness (if
↑doses or RF: reversible).
Interactions: ↑s toxicity of digoxin, aspirin, gentamicin and
lithium. ↓s fx of antidiabetics. NSAIDs may ↓diuretic response.
Monitor: U&Es – if ↓K⁺, try po K⁺ supplements, using ACE-i or
changing to co-amilofruse.
Dose: usually 20–80 mg po/im/iv daily in divided doses. ↑doses
used in acute LVF (see p. 181) and oliguria. If HF or RF, ivi
(max 4 mg/min) can ⇒ smoother control of fluid balance[BNF]. For
blood transfusions, a rough guide is to give 20 mg with every unit if
existing LVF, and with every 2nd unit if *at risk of LVF*.

Give iv if severe peripheral oedema: bowel oedema ⇒ ↓po
absorption.

FYBOGEL

Laxative: bulking agent (ispaghula husk) for constipation (inc IBS).
CI: swallowing difficulties, GI obstruction, faecal impaction,
colonic atony.
Dose: 1 sachet or 10 ml bd after meals with water.

Ensure good hydration, esp if elderly, GI narrowing or ↓GI motility.

GABAPENTIN

Antiepileptic: similar structure to GABA but does not affect GABA
receptors.
Use: neuropathic pain[1], epilepsy[2] (adjunctive Rx of partial
seizures ± 2° generalisation).
Caution: Hx of psychosis or DM, **R/P/B/E**.
SE: fatigue/somnolence, dizziness, cerebellar fx (esp ataxia; see
p. 175), diplopia/amblyopia, headache, rhinitis. Rarely ↓**WCC**,
GI upset, arthralgia/myalgia, skin reactions.
Dose: initially 300 mg od, ↑ing by 300 mg/day to max 1.8 g daily[1]
or 2.4 g daily[2] in 3 divided doses (stop drug over ≥1 wk).

Can give false-positive urinary dipstick results for proteinuria.

GELOFUSINE

Colloid plasma substitute (gelatin-based) for iv fluid resuscitation (see p. 166). 1 l contains 154 mmol Na^+ (but no K^+).

GENTAMICIN

Aminoglycoside: broad-spectrum 'cidal' antibiotic; inhibits ribosomal 30s subunit. Good Gram-negative aerobe/staphylococci cover, otherwise needs concurrent penicillin $\pm$ metronidazole.

Use: severe infections, esp sepsis, meningitis, endocarditis. Also pyelonephritis/prostatitis, biliary tract infections, pneumonia.

CI: MG*.

Caution: obesity, R/P/E (may need to adjust dose).

SE: ototoxic, **nephrotoxic** (dose- and Rx length-dependent), **hypersensitivity**, rash. Rarely AAC, N&V, seizures, encephalopathy, blood disorders, myasthenia-like syndrome* (at ↑d doses; reversible), ↓Mg^{++} (if prolonged Rx).

Monitor: serum levels.

Interactions: fx (esp toxicity) ↑d by loop diuretics (esp **furosemide**), cephalosporins, vancomycin, amphotericin, ciclosporin and cytotoxics; if these drugs must be given, space doses as far from time of gentamicin dose as possible. Anticholinesterase fx are ↓d. Muscle relaxant fx are ↑d.

Dose: 3–5 mg/kg/day in 3 divided doses im/iv/ivi (od regimes possible – contact your pharmacy/microbiology dept for details); 80 mg bd iv for endocarditis Rx.

↓doses if RF (and consider if elderly or ↑↑BMI), otherwise adjust according to serum levels*: call microbiology department if unsure.

Gentamicin levels: measure peak at 1 h post-dose (ideally = 5–10 mg/l) and trough immediately predose (ideally ≤2 mg/l). Halve ideal levels for streptococcal/enterococcal endocarditis. If levels high, can ↑spacing of doses (as well as ↓ing amount of dose); as ⇒ ↑risk of ototoxicity, monitor auditory/vestibular function. NB: different monitoring for od regimes.

GLIBENCLAMIDE

Oral antidiabetic (long-acting sulphonylurea): ↑s pancreatic insulin release – stimulates β islet cell receptors (and inhibits gluconeogenesis).
Use: type 2 DM; requires endogenous insulin to work. Not recommended for obese* (use metformin) or elderly** (use short-acting preparations, e.g. gliclazide).
CI: ketoacidosis, porphyria, **L/R** (if either severe, otherwise caution), **P/B**.
Caution: may need to replace with insulin during intercurrent illness/surgery, **E**.
SE: hypoglycaemia (esp in elderly**), **GI upset**, ↑**Wt***, **headache**. Rarely hypersensitivity (inc skin) reactions, blood disorders, hepatotoxicity.
Interactions: fx ↑d by chloramphenicol, sulphonamides (inc co-trimoxazole), antifungals (esp fluconazole/miconazole), bezafibrate and NSAIDs.
Dose: initially 5 mg mane (with food), ↑ing as necessary (max 15 mg/day).

GLICLAZIDE

Oral antidiabetic (short-acting sulphonylurea).
Use/CI/SE/Interactions: as glibenclamide, but shorter action* and hepatic metabolism** mean ↓d risk of hypoglycaemia (esp in elderly* and RF**).
Dose: initially 40–80 mg mane (with food), ↑ing as necessary (max 320 mg/day).

GLIPIZIDE

Oral antidiabetic (short-acting sulphonylurea).
Use/CI/SE/Interactions: as gliclazide.
Dose: initially 2.5–5.0 mg mane (with food), ↑ing as necessary (max single dose 15 mg; max daily dose 20 mg).

GLUCAGON

Polypeptide hormone: ↑s hepatic glycogen conversion to glucose.

L/R/H = Liver, Renal and Heart failure (full key see p. x)

Use: hypoglycaemia: if acute and severe, esp if no iv access or if 2°
to xs insulin (see p. 188).

CI: phaeo.

Caution: glucagonomas/insulinomas. Will not work if hypoglycaemia is chronic (inc starvation) or 2° to adrenal insufficiency.

SE: N&V&D, ↓BP, ↓K^+, hypersensitivity, **W+**.

Dose: 1 mg (= 1 unit) **im** (or sc/iv).

Often found on crash trolleys.

GLYCEROL (= GLYCERIN) SUPPOSITORIES

Rectal irritant bowel stimulant.

Use: constipation: 1st-line suppository if oral methods such as
lactulose and senna fail.

Dose: 1–2 pr prn.

GLYCERYL TRINITRATE see GTN

GRANISETRON

Antiemetic: $5HT_3$ antagonist.

Use: N&V; see Ondansetron.

Caution: P/B.

SE/Interactions: see Ondansetron.

Dose: 1 mg bd po/iv/ivi for nonspecialist use. 2–3 mg loading doses
often given before chemotherapy[BNF] (max 9 mg/24 h).

GTN (= GLYCERYL TRINITRATE)

Nitrate: ⇒ vasodilation of coronary arteries and systemic veins
⇒ ↑O_2 supply to myocardium and ↓preload, ∴ ↓O_2 demand of
myocardium.

Use: Angina, LVF.

CI: ↓BP, ↓↓Hb, aortic/mitral stenosis, constrictive pericarditis,
tamponade, HOCM, glaucoma (closed-angle).

Caution: recent MI, ↓T_4, hypothermia, head trauma, cerebral
haemorrhage, malnutrition, L/R (if either severe).

SE: ↓BP (inc postural), **headache**, dizziness, flushing, ↑IIR.

Dose: 2 sprays or tablets sl prn (also available as transdermal SR patches[BNF]). For acute MI/LVF: 10–200 µg/min ivi, titrating to clinical response and BP (see p. 178).

HAEMACCEL Colloid plasma substitute (gelatin) used for iv fluid resuscitation (see p. 166). NB: 1 l contains 145 mmol Na^+ and 5.1 mmol K^+.

HALOPERIDOL

Antipsychotic (butyrophenone): blockade of DA ($D_{2\&3} > D_1 > D_4$), and to lesser extent α-adrenergic, $5HT_{2A}$, histamine H_1 and muscarinic receptors.

Use: acute sedation[1] (e.g. agitation, behavioural disturbance – esp in elderly and Ψ disorders), schizophrenia[2], N&V[3].

CI/Caution/SE: as chlorpromazine, but ⇒ ↑incidence of **extrapyramidal fx**, although ⇒ ↓sedation, ↓skin reactions, ↓antimuscarinic fx, ↓BP fx. Rarely neuroleptic malignant syndrome, hypoglycaemia, SIADH.

Interactions: metabolised by P450: fx ↑d by SSRIs, amiodarone, phenytoin, ritonavir and cimetidine.

Dose: 1.5–5.0 mg bd/tds po (max 30 mg/day)[1,2]; 2–10 mg im/iv 4–8-hourly (max 18 mg/day)[1,2]; 0.5–2.0 mg tds im/iv[3]. Also used im as a 'depot'[2]. *Consider ↓ing doses in elderly.*

See pp. 171–2 for practical advice on acute sedation.

HARTMANN'S SOLUTION

Compound sodium lactate iv fluid; used mostly in surgery and trauma. 1 l contains **5 mmol K^+**, 2 mmol Ca^{++}, 29 mmol HCO_3^-, 131 mmol Na^+, 111 mmol Cl^-.

HELICLEAR

Triple-therapy combination preparation of PPI and two antibiotics.

Use: *H. pylori* eradication.

CI/Caution/SE: as per individual drugs.

Dose: lansoprazole 30 mg bd + amoxicillin 1 g bd + clarithromycin 500 mg bd for 7–14 days.

HELIMET as **Heliclear**, but contains metronidazole 400 mg bd instead of amoxicillin 1 g.

HEMINEVRIN see Clomethiazole

HEPARIN, standard/unfractionated (NB: ≠ LMWHs).

iv (and rarely sc) anticoagulant: potentiates protease inhibitor antithrombin III, which inactivates thrombin. Also inhibits factors IXa/Xa/XIa/XIIa.

Use: anticoagulation if needs to be immediate or quickly reversible (only as inpatient); DVT/PE Rx/Px (inc preoperative), MI/unstable angina Rx/Px, extracorporeal circuits (esp haemodialysis, cardiopulmonary bypass).

CI: haemorrhagic disorders (inc haemophilia), ↓Pt (inc Hx of HIT*), severe HTN, PU, recent cerebral haemorrhage or major surgery/trauma (esp eye or nervous system), epidural/spinal anaesthesia (but can give Px doses), **L** (if severe, esp if oesophageal varices).

Caution: ↑K^{+**}, **R/P**.

SE: haemorrhage, ↓Pt* (HIT*), **hypersensitivity** (inc anaphylaxis, urticaria, angioedema), ↑**K**$^{+**}$ (inhibits aldosterone: ↑risk if DM, CRF, acidosis or on K$^+$-sparing drugs), osteoporosis (if prolonged Rx).

Monitor: FBC* if >5 days Rx, U&E** if > 7 days Rx.

Dose: see pp. 159–60 (inc dose-adjustment advice).

> 🔑 HIT* **H**eparin **I**nduced **T**hrombocytopenia: immune mediated ∴ delayed onset – ↑risk if Rx for >5 days (see p. 158). 🔑

HUMALOG see Insulin lispro; short-acting recombinant insulin. Also available as biphasic preparations (**Mix 25**, **Mix 50**) are combined with longer-acting isophane suspension.

HUMULIN recombinant insulin available in various forms:

1 **HUMULIN S** soluble, short-acting for iv/acute use (DKA/sliding scales).
2 **HUMULIN I** isophane (combined with protamine), long-acting.
3 **HUMULIN Lente** insulin zinc suspension, long-acting.

4   HUMULIN Zn crystalline insulin zinc suspension; long-acting.
5   HUMULIN M 'biphasic' preparations, combination of short-acting (S) and long-acting (I) forms to give smoother control throughout the day. Numbers denote 1/10 of the percentage of soluble insulin (i.e. M2 = 20%, M3 = 30%, M5 = 50% soluble insulin).

HYDRALAZINE

Antihypertensive: vasodilates smooth muscle (arteries >veins).
Use: HTN[1] (inc severe[2], esp if RF or pregnancy), HF[3].
CI: severe ↑HR, myocardial insufficiency (2° to mechanical obstruction), cor pulmonale, dissecting aortic aneurysm, SLE*, porphyria, **H** (if high-output).
Caution: IHD, cerebrovascular disease, L/R/P/B.
SE: (all SEs ↓if dose <100 mg/day) ↑**HR, GI upset, headache, lupus-like syndrome*** (watch for unexplained ↓Wt, arthritis, ill health – measure ANA* and dipstick urine for protein if on high doses/clinical suspicion). Also fluid retention (↓d if used with diuretics), palpitations, dizziness, flushing, ↓BP (even at low doses), blood disorders, arthralgia/myalgia.
Dose: 25–50 mg bd po[1]; 5–10 mg iv[2] (can be repeated after 20–30 min) or 50–300 µg/min ivi[2]; 25–75 mg tds/qds po[3].

HYDROCORTISONE BUTYRATE CREAM (0.1%)/
LOCOID
Potent-strength topical corticosteroid. *NB: much stronger than standard (non-butyrate) hydrocortisone cream!*

HYDROCORTISONE CREAM (1%)

Mild-strength topical corticosteroid (rarely used as weaker 0.5%, 0.25% and 0.1% preparations).

HYDROCORTISONE iv/po

Glucocorticoid (mild mineralocorticoid activity).
Use: acute hypersensitivity (esp anaphylaxis, angioedema), Addisonian crisis, asthma, COPD, ↓T[4] (and ↑T[4]), IBD. Also used po in chronic adrenocortical deficiency.

L/R/H = Liver, Renal and Heart failure (full key see p. x)

CI: systemic infection (if no antibiotic cover).
Caution/SE: see pp. 169–70.
Dose: *acutely:* 100–300 mg im or slowly iv. Exact dose recommendations vary: consult local protocol if unsure (see Medical emergencies section of this book for rational starting dose for some specific indications). *Chronic replacement:* usually 20–30 mg po daily in divided doses (usually 2/3 in morning and 1/3 nocte), often together with fludrocortisone.

HYDROXOCOBALAMIN

Vitamin B_{12} replacement.
Use: pernicious anaemia (also macrocytic anaemias with neurological involvement, tobacco amblyopia, Leber's optic atrophy).
SE: skin reactions, GI upset, 'flu-like symptoms, $\downarrow K^+$ (initially), rarely anaphylaxis.
Dose: 1 mg im injection: frequently at first for Rx (3–7/wk: exact number depends on indication[BNF]) until no further improvement, then $\downarrow$frequency (to once every 1–3 months) for maintenance.

HYDROXYCARBAMIDE (= HYDROXYUREA)

Oral agent for CML. 2nd-line Rx for polycythaemia, severe psoriasis.
SE: GI upset, blood disorders (esp **myelosuppression**), skin reactions.
CI/Caution: see product literature.
Dose: 20–30 mg/kg daily (or 80 mg/kg every 3rd day). Specialist use only.

HYOSCINE BUTYLBROMIDE/BUSCOPAN

Antimuscarinic ⇒ $\downarrow$GI motility: does not cross BBB (unlike hyoscine hydrobromide, which is more sedative and effective at controlling secretions).
Use: GI/GU smooth-muscle spasm, esp biliary colic/diverticulitis/IBS (rarely used for dysmenorrhoea).
CI/Caution: see Atropine.
SE: antimuscarinic fx (see p. 174).

Dose: 20 mg qds po (for IBS, start at 10 mg tds) or 20 mg im/iv (repeating once after 30 min, if necessary; can use again under specialist supervision).

Do not confuse with hyoscine hydrobromide: different effects and doses!

HYOSCINE HYDROBROMIDE

Antimuscarinic: predominant fx on CNS (vestibular), ↓s respiratory/oral secretions.

Use: motion sickness[1], terminal care/chronic ↓swallow[2] (e.g. CVA), hypersalivation 2° to antipsychotics[3] (unlicensed use).

CI: glaucoma (closed-angle).

Caution: GI obstruction, ↑prostate/urinary retention, cardio-vascular disease, porphyria, **L/R/P/B/E**.

SE: antimuscarinic fx (see p. 174), generally sedative (but can ⇒ paradoxical agitation when given as sc infusion).

Warn: driving may be impaired, ↑s fx of alcohol.

Dose: 300 µg qds po[1] (or as transdermal patches; release 1 mg over 72 h); 0.6–2.4 mg/24 h as sc infusion[2] (see p. 143 for use in palliative care); 300 µg bd po[3] (can ↑ to qds).

Do not confuse with hyoscine butylbromide: different effects and doses!

HYPROMELLOSE

Artificial tears for Sjogren's/other causes of dry eyes.

Dose: 1–2 drops prn (often given in combination with the mucolytic acetylcysteine for filamentary keratitis).

IBUGEL/IBULEVE ibuprofen topical gel/spray respectively for musculoskeletal pain.

IBUPROFEN

NSAID (propionic acid derivative): unselective COX inhibitor. As well as (mild) anti-inflammatory, it also has antipyrexial and analgesic properties.

Use: mild/moderate pain[1] (headache, gynaecological/musculoskeletal pain; not 1st choice for gout/rheumatoid arthritis), fever[2], mild local inflammation[3].
CI: Hx of hypersensitivity to any NSAID (inc asthma, angioedema, urticaria or rhinitis reactions). Hx of, or active, peptic ulcer*.
Caution: Hx of asthma, GI disease, ↑BP or allergic disorders, L/R/H/P/B/E.
SE: (*generally milder than with other NSAIDs*) **GI upset/ulceration*/bleeding**. Also headache, nervousness, dizziness, fluid retention/oedema, ARF, hypersensitivity reactions (esp bronchospasm and skin reactions, inc SJS/TEN). Rarely, blood disorders, ↑BP.
Interactions: ↓s fx of antihypertensives, ↑s (toxic) fx of methotrexate, AZT, tacrolimus and lithium (mild **W+**).
Dose: 200–400 mg tds po[1&2] (↑dose needed for rheumatoid arthritis: up to 800 mg tds); topically as gel[3].

IMODIUM see Loperamide

INDAPAMIDE
Thiazide derivative diuretic.
Use: HTN.
CI: recent CVA, **L** (if severe).
Caution: hyperparathyroidism, R/P/B/E.
SE: as bendroflumethiazide, but reportedly fewer metabolic disturbances (esp less hyperglycaemia).
Monitor: U&Es, urate.
Interactions: ↑s lithium levels.
Dose: 2.5 mg od mane (or 1.5 mg od of SR preparation).

INDOMETACIN
High-strength NSAID; unselective COX inhibitor.
Use: musculoskeletal pain[1]; esp gout, ankylosing spondylitis, rheumatoid arthritis, dysmennorhoea (use limited by SEs*). Also used in specialist setting for PDA closure.
CI/Caution/SE: as ibuprofen, but ↑incidence of SEs, esp GI bleeding, headaches, dizziness, Ψ disturbances (dose-dependent).

Dose: 25–50 mg up to qds po or 100 mg up to bd pr (max total daily dose 200 mg)[1]. Use high doses initially for gout, and ↓dose once pain under control. SR preparations available[BNF] (75–200 mg/day in 1–2 divided doses).

▼INFLIXIMAB/REMICADE

Monoclonal Ab against TNF-α (inflammatory cytokine).
Use: Crohn's disease, rheumatoid arthritis or ankylosing spondylitis resistant to steroids/immunosuppression[NICE].
CI: TB or other severe infections, **H/P/B**.
SE: severe infections, TB (inc extrapulmonary), **CCF** (exac of), **CNS demyelination**. Also GI upset, 'flu-like symptoms, cough, fatigue, headache. ↑incidence of hypersensitivity (esp transfusion) reactions.
Dose: specialist use only.

INSULATARD long-acting (isophane) insulin, either recombinant human or porcine.

INSULIN see pp. 150–4 for different types and prescribing advice.

INTEGRILIN see Eptifibatide; anti-Pt agent for IHD.

IPOCOL see Mesalazine; 'new' aminosalicylate for UC, with ↓SEs.

IPRATROPIUM

Inh muscarinic antagonist: ⇒ bronchodilation, ↓s bronchial secretions.
Use: chronic[1] and acute[2] bronchospasm (COPD >asthma). Rarely used topically for rhinitis.
SE: antimuscarinic fx (see p. 174), usually minimal.
Caution: glaucoma (protect patient's eyes from drug, esp if giving nebs: use tight-fitting mask), bladder outflow obstruction (e.g. ↑prostate), **P/B**.
Dose: 20–80 μg qds inh[1]; 250–500 μg qds neb[2] (↑ing up to 4-hourly if severe).

IRBESARTAN/APROVEL

Angiotensin II antagonist.

Use: HTN, type 2 DM nephropathy.
CI: P/B.
Caution/SE/Interactions: see Losartan.
Dose: initially 150 mg od, ↑ing to 300 mg od if required (halve initial dose if age >75 years or on haemodialysis).

IRON TABLETS see Ferrous sulphate

ISDN see Isosorbide dinitrate

ISMN see Isosorbide mononitrate

ISMO see Isosorbide mononitrate

ISONIAZID

Antibiotic, 'cidal'.
Use: TB (see p. 131).
CI: L (if drug-induced).
Caution: Hx of psychosis/epilepsy/porphyria or if ↑d risk of neuritis (e.g. DM, alcohol abuse, CRF, malnutrition, HIV: give pyridoxine 10–20 mg od as Px), porphyria, **L/R/P/B**.
SE: optic neuritis, **peripheral neuropathy**, **hepatitis***, rash, gynaecomastia, GI upset. Rarely lupus, blood disorders, hypersensitivity, convulsions, psychosis.
Warn: patient of symptoms of liver disease and to seek medical help if they occur.
Monitor: LFTs*, FBC.
Interactions: ↓P450 ∴ many, but most importantly ↑s levels of carbamazepine, phenytoin and benzodiazepines, **W+**.
Dose: by weight^BNF or as combination preparation (see p. 131). Take on empty stomach (≥30 min before or ≥2 h after meal).
Acetylator-dependent metabolism: if slow acetylator ⇒ ↑risk of SEs.

ISOSORBIDE DINITRATE (ISDN)

Nitrate.
Use/CI/Caution/SE: as GTN, but also available as po preparations (also ⇒ ↓headache).

Dose: 5–10 mg sl prn; 10–80 mg tds po, titrating up slowly (bd MR preparations available[BNF]); 2–20 mg/h ivi (write up exactly the same as for GTN on p. 178, i.e. 50 mg made up to 50 ml at 0–10 ml/h).

Sublingual preparations of ISDN are more stable over time than those of GTN and ∴ better for those who need nitrates infrequently (less drug ends up being thrown away!)

ISOSORBIDE MONONITRATE (ISMN)

Nitrate.
Use/Cl/Caution/SE: as GTN, but *available only as po preparations*.
Dose: 10–40 mg bd/tds po (od MR preparations available[BNF]).

ISTIN see Amlodipine

ITRACONAZOLE/SPORANOX

Triazole antifungal: needs acidic pH for good po absorption*.
Use: fungal infections (candida, tinea, cryptococcus, aspergillosis, histoplasmosis, onychomycosis, pityriasis versicolor).
Caution: risk of HF: Hx of cardiac disease or if on negative inotropic drugs (risk ↑s w dose, length of Rx and age), **L/R/P/B**.
SE: HF, hepatotoxicity, **GI upset**, **headache**, dizziness, peripheral neuropathy (if occurs, stop drug), cholestasis, menstrual Δs, skin reactions (inc angioedema, SJS). With prolonged Rx, ↓K+, oedema, hair loss.
Monitor: LFTs** if Rx >1 month or Hx of (or develop clinical features of) liver disease: stop drug if become abnormal.
Interactions: ↓**P450** ∴ many; most importantly ↑s risk of **myopathy with statins** (avoid together) and ↑s risk of **HF with negative inotropes** (esp Ca++ blockers). ↑s fx of digoxin, quinidine, indinavir, midazolam, ciclosporin and sirolimus/tacrolimus. fx ↓d by rifampicin, phenytoin and **antacids***, **W+**.
Dose: dependent on indication[BNF]. *Take with food.*

KAY-CEE-L
KCl syrup (1 mmol/ml).

Use: ↓K⁺.
CI/Caution/SE: as Sando-K.
Dose: according to serum K⁺: average 25–50 ml/day if diet normal
(↓ if renal impairment).

KETOCONAZOLE/NIZORAL

Imidazole antifungal: good po absorption.
Use: fungal infections (if systemic, severe or resistant to topical Rx),
Px if immunosuppression.
CI: L/P/B.
Caution: porphyria.
SE: ☻ hepatitis* ☠, **GI upset**, **skin reactions** (rash, urticaria,
pruritus, photosensitivity, rarely angioedema), **gynaecomastia**,
blood disorders, paraesthesia, dizziness, photophobia.
Monitor: LFTs*, esp if Rx >14 days.
Interactions: ↓**P450** ∴ many; most importantly, ↑s risk of
myopathy with statins (avoid together). ↑s fx of midazolam, indinavir
and ciclosporin (and possibly theophyllines). ↓s fx of rifampicin
(rifampicin can also ↓ fx of ketoconazole, as can phenytoin), **W+**.
Dose: 200 mg od po *with food* (400 mg od in severe/resistant
infections).

KLEAN-PREP see Bowel preparations
Dose: up to 2 powder sachets the evening before and repeated on
the morning of GI surgery or Ix.

KLOREF
Effervescent oral KCl (6.7 mmol K⁺/tablet).
Use: ↓K⁺.
CI/Caution/SE: as Sando-K.
Dose: according to serum K⁺: average 4–8 tablets/day if diet
normal (↓ if renal impairment).

LABETALOL

β-blocker with arteriolar vasodilatory properties ∴ also ⇒ ↓TPR.
Use: severe HTN (inc during pregnancy[1] or post-MI[2]).

CI/Caution/SE: as propranolol, plus can ⇒ ☠ **severe/postural** ↓**BP** ☠ and hepatotoxicity* (L).

Monitor: LFTs (if deteriorate stop drug).

Dose: initially 100 mg bd po (halve dose in elderly), ↑ing every fortnight if necessary to max of 600 mg qds po; if essential to ↓BP rapidly give 50 mg iv over ≥ 1 min repeating after 5 min if necessary (or can give 2 mg/min ivi), up to max total dose 200 mg; 20 mg/h ivi[1], doubling every 30 min to max of 160 mg/h; 15 mg/h ivi[2], ↑ing slowly to max of 120 mg/h.

LACRI-LUBE

Artificial tears for dry eyes.

SE: blurred vision.

Dose: 1–2 drops prn (best used nocte).

LACTULOSE

Osmotic laxative[1]: semisynthetic disaccharide bulking agent. Also ↓s growth of NH_4-producing bacteria[2].

Use: constipation[1], hepatic encephalopathy[2].

CI: GI obstruction, galactosaemia.

SE: flatulence, distension, abdominal pains.

Dose: 10–15 ml bd[1] (↑dose according to response; NB: *can take 2 days to work*); 30–50 ml tds[2].

LAMOTRIGINE/LAMICTAL

Antiepileptic: ↓s release of excitatory amino acids (esp glutamate) via action on voltage-sensitive Na^+ channels

Use: epilepsy (esp partial, 1°/2° generalised tonic-clonic).

Caution: avoid abrupt withdrawal, L/R/P/B/E.

SE: cerebellar symptoms (see p. 175), **skin reactions*** (often severe, e.g. SJS, TEN, lupus, esp in children or if also on valproate), **blood disorders**** (↓Hb, ↓WCC, ↓Pt), N&V. Rarely, ↓memory, sedation, Ψ disorders, sleep Δ, acne, pretibial ulcers, alopecia, worsening of seizures, polyuria/anuria, **hepatotoxicity**.

Monitor: U&Es, FBC, LFTs, clotting.

Warn: report rash*, 'flu-like symptoms, signs of infection/↓Hb, bruising**.

Interactions: fx are ↓d by phenytoin, carbamazepine. fx ↑d by valproate.
Dose: 25–700 mg daily^{BNF} (↑dose slowly to ↓risk of skin reactions).

LANSOPRAZOLE/ZOTON
PPI. As omeprazole, but ↓ interactions.
Dose: 30 mg od po (↓ to 15 mg od for maintenance).

LARIAM see Mefloquine

LATANOPROST/XALATAN
Topical PG analogue: ↑s uveoscleral outflow.
Use: glaucoma: if refractory open-angle, 2° causes or refractory *ocular* HTN.
Caution: asthma (if severe), aphakia, pseudophakia, **P/B**.
SE: blurred vision, local reactions, ↑s brown pigmentation of iris (in green/brown irides). Rarely cystoid macular oedema, uveitis, angina.
Dose: 1 drop od (nocte) of 50-μg/ml solution.

LASIX see Furosemide

▼LEFLUNOMIDE/ARAVA
DMARD; inhibits pyrimidine synthesis (also anti-inflammatory fx).
Use: moderate/severe active rheumatoid arthritis if standard DMARDs (e.g. methotrexate or sulfasalazine) CI or not tolerated.
CI: severe immunodeficiency, BM suppression, hypoproteinaemia, serious infection, **L/R/P/B**.
Caution: blood disorders, TB (inc Hx of).
SE: BM toxicity, ↑risk of **infection/malignancy,** hepatotoxicity, HTN.
Warn: teratogenic: must exclude pregnancy before starting Rx and use contraception during Rx (and until drug no longer active*).
Monitor: LFTs, FBC, BP.
Dose: specialist use only.

Long $t_{1/2}$*: needs prolonged washout period or active measures (e.g. cholestyramine 8 g tds or activated charcoal 50 g qds) to ↑elimination if wishing to conceive.

LEVOBUNOLOL

β-blocker eye drops: similar to timolol ⇒ ↓aqueous humour production. *Significant systemic absorption can occur.*

Use: chronic simple glaucoma.

CI: ↓HR, HB, uncontrolled HF, asthma/COPD.

SE: local reactions. Rarely anterior uveitis, anaphylaxis, broncho-constriction, cardiac fx (see Propranolol).

Interactions: as propranolol (esp **verapamil**).

Dose: 1 drop of 0.5% solution od/bd.

LEVODOPA (= L-DOPA)

Precursor of dopamine: needs concomitant peripheral dopa decarboxylase inhibitor such as benserazide (see Co-beneldopa) or carbidopa (see Co-careldopa) to limit SEs.

Use: parkinsonism.

CI: glaucoma (closed-angle), **P/B**.

Caution: pulmonary/cardiovascular/Ψ disease, melanoma (can reactivate), DM, osteomalacia, PU, **L/R**.

SE: dyskinesias, **abdominal upset**, **postural** ↓BP, **drowsiness**, **aggression**, **Ψ disorders** (confusion, depression, suicide, hallucinations, psychosis, hypomania), seizures, dizziness, headache, flushing, sweating, peripheral neuropathy, taste Δs, rash/prutitus, Δ LFTs, GI bleeding, blood disorders, dark body fluids (inc sweat).

Warn: daytime sleepiness.

Interactions: fx ↓d by neuroleptics, SEs ↑d by bupropion, **risk of ↑BP crisis with MAOIs**, risk of arrhythmias with halothane.

Dose: 125–500 mg daily, *after food*, ↑ing according to response.

Abrupt withdrawal can ⇒ neuroleptic malignant-like syndrome.

LEVOTHYROXINE see Thyroxine

LEVOMEPROMAZINE (= METHOTRIMEPRAZINE)/ NOZINAN

Phenothiazine: antipsychotic, **antiemetic**: acts on multiple receptors (as chlorpromazine, but ↑muscarinic/α blockade).

Use: N&V[1] (esp if resistant to standard Rx), rarely schizophrenia.

CI/Caution/SE/Interactions: as chlorpromazine, but ↑incidence of postural ↓**BP** (esp in elderly: do not give if age >50 years and ambulant).
Dose: 12.5–25 mg im/iv tds/qds[1], or 25–200 mg/24 h sc infusion[1]; see p. 143 for use in palliative care. *Lower doses may be effective and ⇒ ↓sedation.*

LIBRIUM see Chlordiazepoxide

LIDOCAINE (previously LIGNOCAINE)

Class Ib antiarrhythmic (slows conduction in Purkinje and ventricular muscle fibres), local anaesthetic (blocks fast Na^+ channels in axons).
Use: ventricular arrhythmias (esp VT and post-MI). Also local anaesthesia.
CI: myocardial depression (if severe), SAN disorders, atrio-ventricular block, porphyria.
Caution: epilesy, **L/H/E**.
SE: **dizziness, drowsiness, confusion, tinnitus,** blurred vision, paraesthesia, GI upset, arrhythmias, ↓BP, ↓HR. Rarely respiratory depression, seizures, hypersensitivity.
Monitor: ECG during iv administration.
Dose (for *arrhythmias*): 50–100 mg iv over 1–2 min followed immediately by ivi at 4 mg/min for 30 min then 2 mg/min for 2 h and 1 mg/min thereafter (↓dose further if drug needed for >24 h). If >15 min delay in setting up ivi, can give max 2 further doses of 50–100 mg iv ≥ 10 min apart. In emergencies, can often be found stocked in crash trolleys as Minijet syringes of 1% (10 mg/ml) or 2% (20 mg/ml) solutions. *For use in ALS Broad complex tachycardia algorithm see inside front cover.*

☠ Local anaesthetic preparations must never be injected into veins or inflamed tissue, as can ⇒ systemic fx (esp arrhythmias). ☠

LIGNOCAINE see Lidocaine

LIOTHYRONINE (SODIUM) (= T_3)

Synthetic T_3: quicker and more potent action than thyroxine (T_4).

Use: acute hypothyroidism (e.g. myxoedema coma*: see p. 189).
CI/Caution/SE: see Thyroxine.
Dose: 5–20 µg iv slowly. Repeat every 4–12 h as necessary; seek
expert help. Also available po, but thyroxine (T_4) preferred for
maintenance use.

Concurrent hydrocortisone iv is often also needed*; see p. 189.

LISINOPRIL

ACE-i; see Captopril.
Use: HTN[1], HF[2], Px of IHD post-MI[3], DM nephropathy[4].
CI/Caution/SE: as captopril.
Dose: initially 2.5 mg od[1,2,4], ↑ing if necessary (maintenance usually
5–20 mg daily; max 40 mg/day). Doses post-MI depend on BP[BNF].

LITHIUM

Mood stabiliser: inhibits inositol phosphate/cAMP 2nd-messenger
systems. Competes with other anions at Na^+/K^+ pump, changing
tissue cation exchange.
Use: mania Rx/Px, bipolar disorder Px (rarely for recurrent
depression Px).
CI: ↓T_4 (if untreated), Addison's, SSS, cardiovascular disease,
P (⇒ Ebstein's anomaly: esp in 1st trimester), **R/H/B**.
(NB: manufacturers don't agree on definitive list and all CI are
relative – decisions should be made in clinical context and expert
help sought if unsure.)
Caution: thyroid disease, MG, E.
SE: thirst, polyuria, GI upset (↑Wt, N&V&D), fine tremor*, tardive
dyskinesia, muscular weakness, acne. Rarer but serious: ↓T_4 (esp in
females ± goitre), renal impairment (diabetes insipidus, interstitial
nephritis), arrhythmias.
Monitor: serum levels 12 h post-*Dose:* keep at 0.4–1.0 mmol/l
(>1.5 mmol/l may ⇒ toxicity, esp if elderly), U&Es, TFTs.
Warn: report symptoms of ↓T_4, avoid dehydration.
Interactions: toxicity (± levels) ↑d by NSAIDs, SSRIs, ACE-i,
diuretics** (esp thiazides), methyldopa and antipsychotics.
Theophyllines, caffeine and antacids may ↓ lithium levels.

L/R/H = Liver, **R**enal and **H**eart failure (full key see p. x)

Dose: see BNF/product literature: 2 *types* (salts) available with different doses ('carbonate' 200 mg = 'citrate' 509 mg) and bioavailabilities of particular *brands* vary ∴ *must specify salt and brand required.*

Consider stopping 24 h before major surgery; restart once electrolytes return to normal.

Lithium toxicity

Features: D&V, coarse tremor*, cerebellar signs (see p. 00), renal impairment/oliguria, ↓BP, ↑reflexes, convulsions, drowsiness ⇒ coma. *Rx:* stop drug, control seizures, correct electrolytes (normally need saline ivi; high risk if ↓Na^+: avoid low-salt diets and diuretics**). Consider haemodialysis if RF.

LOCOID see Hydrocortisone butyrate 0.1% (potent steroid) cream

LOPERAMIDE/IMODIUM

Antimotility agent: synthetic opioid analogue; binds to receptors in GI muscle ⇒ ↓peristalsis, ↑transit time, ↑H_2O/electrolyte resorption, ↓gut secretions, ↑sphincter tone. Extensive 1st-pass metabolism ⇒ minimal systemic opioid fx.

Use: diarrhoea.

CI: constipation, ileus, abdominal distension, active UC/AAC.

Caution: in young (can ⇒ fluid + electrolyte depletion), L/P.

SE: constipation, abdominal cramps, bloating, dizziness, drowsiness, fatigue. Rarely hypersensitivity (esp skin reactions), paralytic ileus.

Dose: initially 4 mg, then 2 mg after each loose stool (max 16 mg/day for 5 days).

LORATADINE

Non-sedating antihistamine: see Cetirizine.

Dose: 10 mg od. Non-proprietary or as Clarityn.

LORAZEPAM

Benzodiazepine, short-acting.

Use: sedation[1] (esp acute behavioural disturbance/Ψ disorders, e.g. acute psychosis), status epilepticus[2].

CI/Caution/SE/Interactions: see Diazepam.
Dose: 0.5–2 mg po/im/iv prn (bottom of this range if elderly/
respiratory disease/naive to benzodiazepines; top of range if young/
recent exposure to benzodiazepines; max 4 mg/day)[1]; 0.1 mg/kg ivi
at 2 mg/min[2].

☠ Beware respiratory depression: have flumazenil and O_2
(± resuscitation trolley) at hand, esp if respiratory disease or
giving high doses im/iv. ☠

LOSARTAN/COZAAR

Angiotensin II antagonist: specifically blocks renin–angiotensin
system ∴ does not inhibit bradykinin and ⇒ dry cough.
Use: HTN, Px of type 2 DM nephropathy (if ACE-i not tolerated*).
CI: P/B.
Caution: RAS, HOCM, mitral/aortic stenosis, **L/R/E**.
SE/Interactions: as captopril, but ↓dry cough (major reason for
ACE-i intolerance*). As with ACE-i, can ⇒ ↑K^+ (esp if taking ↑K^+-
sparing diuretics/salt substitutes or if RF).
Dose: initially 25–50 mg od (↑ing to max 100 mg od).

LOSEC see Omeprazole

LUGOL'S SOLUTION

Oral I_2 solution.
Use: ↑T_4 if severe ('thyroid storm' see pp. 188–9) or pre-operatively.
CI: B.
Caution: not for long-term Rx, P.
SE: hypersensitivity.
Dose: 0.1–0.3 ml tds (of solution containing 130 mg iodine/ml).

MAGNESIUM SULPHATE (iv)

Mg^{++} replacement.
Use: life-threatening asthma[1], serious arrhythmias[2] (esp if torsades
or if ↓K^+; often caused by ↓Mg^{++}), MI[3] (equivocal evidence of
↓mortality), eclampsia[4] (↓s seizures), symptomatic ↓Mg^{++}[5]
(mostly 2° to GI loss).
Caution: L/R.

SE: flushing, ↓BP, GI upset, thirst, ↓reflexes, weakness, confusion/drowsiness. Rarely arrhythmias, respiratory depression, coma.
Dose: 8 mmol ivi over 20 min[1]; 8 mmol ivi over 10–15 min[2] (repeating once if required); 8 mmol ivi over 20 min then ivi of 65–72 mmol over 24 h[3]; see BNF[4]; up to 160 mmol iv/im according to need[5] (over up to 5 days). Available as 50% solution (= 2 mmol/ml = 0.5 g/ml); must dilute 1 part with ⩾1.5 parts water for injection.

MANNITOL
Osmotic diuretic.
Use: cerebral oedema[1] (and glaucoma).
CI: pulmonary oedema, **H**.
SE: GI upset, fever/chills, oedema. Rarely seizures, **H**.
Dose: 1 g/kg (= 5 ml/kg of 20% solution) as rapid ivi[1].

MAXOLON see Metoclopramide

MEBEVERINE
Antispasmodic: direct action on GI muscle.
Use: GI smooth-muscle cramps (esp IBS, diverticulitis).
CI: ileus (paralytic).
Caution: porphyria, **P/B**.
SE: hypersensitivity/skin reactions.
Dose: 135–150 mg tds (20 min before food) or 200 mg bd of SR preparation (Colofac MR).

MEFENAMIC ACID/PONSTAN
Mild NSAID; unselective COX inhibitor.
Use: musculoskeletal pain, esp dysmenorrhoea (also used for menorrhagia).
CI/Caution/SE: as ibuprofen, but also CI if IBD, caution if porphyria and can ⇒ severe diarrhoea, skin reactions, blood disorders (esp haemolytic ↓Hb, ↓Pt); stop drug if suspect. **W+**.
Dose: 500 mg tds po.

MEFLOQUINE/LARIAM
Antimalarial.

Use: malaria Px[1] (in areas of chloroquine-resistant falciparum spp) and Rx[2] (if falciparum spp known or suspected *and not taking the drug as Px*).

CI: hypersensitivity (inc to *quinine*), Hx of neuro-Ψ disorders (inc depression, convulsions).

Caution: epilepsy, cardiac conduction disorders, L/P/B.

SE: GI upset, neuro-Ψ reactions (dizziness, ↓balance, headache, convulsions, sleep disorders, neuropathies, tremor, anxiety, depression, psychosis, hallucinations, panic attacks, agitation). Also cardiac fx (AV block, other conduction disorders, ↑ or ↓HR, ↑ or ↓BP), hypersensitivity reactions.

Warn: patient of neuro-Ψ reactions, start Px 2–3 wks before travel to identify adverse reactions (75% of reactions occur by 3rd dose).

Dose: 250 mg once-weekly[1] (↓dose if Wt <45 kg[BNF]). See BNF[2].

MESALAZINE

'New' aminosalicylate: as sulfasalazine, but with ↓sulphonamide SEs.

Use: UC (Rx/maintenance of remission).

CI: *hypersensitivity to any salicylates,* coagulopathies, **R** (unless mild), **L** (if severe).

Caution: P/B/E.

SE: GI upset, blood disorders, hypersensitivity (inc **lupus**), RF.

Dose: as Asacol (or Ipocol, Pentasa or Salofalk).

MESNA

Binds to metabolite (acreolin) of thiol-containing chemotherapy agents (cyclophosphamide, ifosamide, oxazaphosphorines), which is toxic to urothelium and can ⇒ severe haemorrhagic cystitis. Give as Px before chemotherapy; see product literature for details.

METFORMIN

Oral antidiabetic (biguanide): ⇒ ↑insulin sensitivity w/o affecting levels (⇒ ↓gluconeogenesis and ↓GI absorption of glucose and ↑peripheral use of glucose). Only active in presence of endogenous insulin (i.e. functional islet cells).

Use: type 2 DM: usually 1st-line if diet control unsuccessful (esp if obese, as ⇒ less ↑Wt cf sulphonylureas).

CI: DKA, ↑risk of lactic acidosis (e.g. severe dehydration/infection/ peripheral vascular disease, shock, major trauma, respiratory failure, alcohol dependence, **recent MI***/**X-ray contrast media***), **L/R/P/B**.
SE: GI upset (esp initially and with ↑doses), metallic taste, headache. Rarely ↓vitamin B_{12} absorption, lactic acidosis.
Dose: initially 500 mg mane, ↑ing as required to max 3 g/day usually in 2 or 3 divided doses. *Take with meals.*

☠ *Both often coexist in coronary angiography: stop drug on day of procedure (giving insulin if necessary; see pp. 150–4) and restart 48 h later, having checked that renal function has not deteriorated. ☠

METHADONE

Opioid agonist: ameliorates opiate withdrawal symptoms.
Use: opioid dependence.
CI/Caution/SE: see Morphine.
Dose: *individual requirements vary widely according to level of previous abuse:* sensible starting dose is 10–20 mg/day po, ↑ing by 10–20 mg every day until no signs or symptoms of withdrawal – which usually stop at 40–60 mg/day. Then aim to wean off gradually. Available as non-proprietary solutions (1 mg/ml) or as Methadose (10 mg/ml or 20 mg/ml). Can give sc/im[BNF].

☠ Do not confuse solutions of different strengths. ☠

METHIONINE

Sulphur-containing amino acid: binds toxic metabolites of paracetamol.
Use: paracetamol OD *<12 h post-ingestion* (ineffective after this), mostly when acetylcysteine ivi cannot be given (e.g. outside hospital).
Caution: L.
SE: N&V, irritability, drowsiness.
Dose: 2.5 g po 4-hourly (for *4 doses only: total dose = 10 g*).

METHOTREXATE

Immunosuppressant, antimetabolite: dihydrofolate reductase inhibitor (↓s nucleic acid synthesis).
Use: rheumatoid arthritis[1] (1st line DMARD), **psoriasis** (if severe/ resistant), **Ca** (ALL, non-Hodgkin's lymphoma, choriocarcinoma, various solid tumours), rarely in Crohn's disease.

CI: severe blood disorders, active infections, immunodeficiency, **R** (if severe), **L** (inc recent hepatitis), **P/B**.

Caution: effusions (esp ascites and pleural effusions: accumulates and returns to blood ⇒ ↑toxicity), blood disorders, UC, PU, ↓immunity, porphyria, **E**.

SE: mucositis/GI upset, myelosuppression, skin reactions. Rarely **pulmonary fibrosis/ pneumonitis** (esp in rheumatoid arthritis), hepatotoxicity, neurotoxicity (inc necrotising demyelinating leukoencephalopathy), seizures, RF (esp tubular necrosis).

Monitor: U&Es, FBC, LFTs.

Interactions: NSAIDs*, corticosteroids, probenecid, **trimethoprim, co-trimoxazole**, penicillins, tetracyclines, chloramphenicol, omeprazole and ciclosporin all ⇒ ↑toxicity.

Warn: avoid over-the-counter NSAIDs*, report any clinical features of infection (esp sore throat).

Dose: 7.5 mg **once a week**[1] (can split dose into 3 × 2.5 mg at 12-h intervals), max 20 mg/wk. For other uses see BNF/product literature.
☠NB: dose is only once a week: potentially fatal if given daily. ☠

METHOTRIMEPRAZINE see Levomepromazine

METHYLDOPA

Centrally acting α_2 agonist.

Use: HTN, esp pregnancy-induced and for essential HTN during pregnancy.

CI: depression, phaeo, porphyria, **L**.

Caution: Hx of depression, **R**.

SE: (minimal if dose <1 g/day) dry mouth, sedation, dizziness, weakness, headache, GI upset, postural ↓BP, ↓HR. Rarely **blood disorders, hepatotoxicity**, pancreatitis, Ψ disorders, parkinsonism.

Monitor: FBC, LFTs.

Interactions: ↑s neurotoxicity of lithium. Hypotensive fx ↑d by antidepressants, anaesthetics and salbutamol ivi.

Dose: initially 250 mg bd/tds (125 mg bd in elderly), ↑ing gradually on alternate days to max of 3 g/day.

METHYLPREDNISOLONE

Glucocorticoid (mild mineralocorticoid activity).

Use: acute flares of inflammatory diseases[1] (esp rheumatoid arthritis, MS), cerebral oedema, Rx of graft rejection.

CI/Caution/SE: see Prednisolone and steroids section (pp. 169–71).

Dose: acutely, up to 1 g ivi od[1] (normally for 3 days). Also available po and as im depot.

METOCLOPRAMIDE/MAXOLON

Antiemetic: D_2 antagonist: acts on central chemoreceptor trigger zone and directly stimulates GI tract ($\Rightarrow$ ↑motility).

Use: N&V, esp GI (gastroduodenal, biliary, hepatic) or opiate-/chemotherapy-induced.

CI: GI obstruction/perforation/haemorrhage (inc 3–4 days post-GI surgery), phaeo, **B**.

Caution: epilepsy, porphyria, L/R/P/E.

SE: extrapyramidal fx (esp in elderly and young females: reversible if drug stopped w/in 24 h or with procyclidine), **drowsiness**, restlessness, GI upset, behavioural/mood Δs, ↑prolactin. Rarely skin reactions, neuroleptic malignant syndrome.

Interactions: ↑s fx of NSAIDs and ciclosporin levels. ↑s risk of extrapyramidal fx of antipsychotics, SSRIs and TCAs.

Dose: 10 mg tds po/im/iv.

METOLAZONE

Potent thiazide-like diuretic: as bendroflumethiazide, plus has additive diuretic fx with loop diuretics.

Use: oedema[1], HTN.

CI/Caution/SE: see Bendroflumethiazide.

Dose: 5–10 mg od po (mane), ↑ing if needed to max of 80 mg/day[1].

METOPROLOL

β-blocker, cardioselective ($\beta_1 > \beta_2$), short-acting.

Use: HTN[1], angina[2], arrhythmias[3], migraine Px[4], ↑T4 (adjunct)[5].

CI/Caution/SE: see Propranolol.

Dose: 50–100 mg bd[1,4]; 50–100 mg bd/tds[2,3]; 50 mg qds[5]. Can give iv[BNF]. See p. 179 for use in AMI/ACS.

METRONIDAZOLE/FLAGYL

Antibiotic, 'cidal': binds DNA of anaerobic and microaerophilic bacteria.

Use: anaerobic and protozoal infections, abdominal sepsis (esp bacteroides), aspiration pneumonia, *C. difficile* (AAC), *H. pylori* eradication (see p. 133), giardia/entamoeba infections, Px during GI surgery. Also dental/gynaecological infections, bacterial vaginosis (*Gardnerella*), PID.

Caution: avoid with alcohol: drug metabolised to acetaldehyde and other toxins ⇒ flushing, abdominal pain, ↓BP (= disulfiram-like reaction), **L/P/B**.

SE: GI upset (esp N&V), metallic taste, skin reactions. Rarely, drowsiness, headache, dizziness, dark urine, hepatotoxicity, blood disorders, myalgia, arthralgia, seizures (transient), ataxia, **peripheral neuropathy** (if prolonged Rx).

Interactions: can ↑lithium/phenytoin levels, **W+**.

Dose: 500 mg tds po/iv for severe infections. Lower doses can be given po (using 200-mg or 400-mg tablets) or higher doses pr (1 g bd/tds) according to indication[BNF].

surg ~ i.v. →po = 400 mg TDS

MICONAZOLE/DAKTARIN

Imidazole antifungal (topical) but *significant systemic absorption can occur.*

Use: oral fungal infections.

CI: L.

Caution: porphyria, **P/B**.

SE: GI upset. Rarely hypersensitivity, hepatotoxicity.

Interactions: as ketoconazole, but rarer. **W+**.

Dose: oral gel 5–10 ml qds (after food).

MIDAZOLAM

Benzodiazepine, very short-acting.

Use: sedation for stressful/painful procedures (esp if amnesia desirable).

CI/Caution/SE/Interactions: see Diazepam.

L/R/H = Liver, Renal and Heart failure (full key see p. x)

Dose: 1.0–7.5 mg iv (titrate up slowly until desired sedation achieved using 0.5–1.0-mg boluses). Can aslo give im[BNF].

☠ Beware respiratory depression: have flumazenil and O_2 (± resuscitation trolley) at hand, esp if respiratory disease or giving high doses im/iv. ☠

MINOCYCLINE

Tetracycline antibiotic: inhibits ribosomal (30S subunit) protein synthesis; broadest spectrum of tetracyclines.

Use: acne.

CI/Caution/SE/Interactions: as tetracycline, but ↓bacterial resistance, although ↑risk of SLE and irreversible skin/body fluid discoloration. Can also use (with caution) in RF.

Dose: 100 mg bd po (or 100 mg od of MR preparation).

MINOXIDIL

Peripheral vasodilator (arterioles ≫ veins): also ⇒ ↑CO, ↑HR, fluid retention ∴ *always needs concurrent β-blocker and diuretic*.

Use: HTN (if severe and Rx-resistant).

CI: phaeo.

Caution: IHD, porphyria, R/P/B.

SE: hypertrichosis, coarsening of facial features (reversible, but makes it *unsuitable for women*), ↑Wt, peripheral oedema, pericardial effusions, angina (dt ↑HR). Rarely, GI upset, gynaecomastia/breast tenderness, renal impairment, skin reactions.

Dose: initially 2.5–5 mg/day in 1 or 2 divided doses, ↑ing if needed up to max of 50 mg/day (↓dose in elderly and dialysis patients). Also used topically for male-pattern baldness.

MIRTAZAPINE/ZISPIN

Antidepressant: **N**oradrenaline **A**nd **S**pecific **S**erotonin **A**gonist (NASSA); specifically stimulates $5HT_1$ receptors (antagonises $5HT_2/5HT_3$), antagonises central presynaptic α_2 receptors.

Use: depression (esp in elderly[*]).

CI/Caution/SE: similar to fluoxetine. Also ⇒ **less sexual dysfunction** and ↓GI upset, although ⇒ ↑**sedation** and ↑**appetite/Wt** (although

both can be beneficial in elderly*). Rarely, blood disorders (inc agranulocytosis**), Δ LFTs, convulsions, myoclonus, oedema.
Warn: patient to report signs of infection** (esp sore throat, fever): stop drug and check FBC if concerned.
Interactions: avoid with other sedatives (inc alcohol). ☠Never give with MAOIs.☠
Dose: initially 15 mg nocte (max 45 mg/day).

MISOPROSTOL
PGE$_1$ analogue: ↓s gastric secretions.
Use: Rx/Px of PU (esp NSAID-induced). Also unlicensed use for induction of medical abortion and ripening cervix for surgical abortion.
CI: ☠pregnancy☠(actual or planned), **B**.
Caution: cardiovascular/cerebrovascular disease.
SE: diarrhoea. Rarely, other GI upset, menstrual Δs, uterine pains.
Dose: most often used with diclofenac as Arthrotec. (Also available with naproxen.)

MIXTARD "biphasic" insulin preparations, available as 20, 30, 40 or 50, which refer to the percentage of soluble (short-acting) insulin; the rest is isophane (long-lasting) insulin.

MMF see Mycophenolate mofetil

MONTELUKAST/SINGULAIR
Leukotriene receptor antagonist: ↓s Ag-induced bronchoconstriction.
Use: *non-acute* asthma (see BTS guidelines, p. 139), esp if large exercise-induced component.
Caution: acute asthma, Churg-Strauss syndrome **P/B**.
SE: headache, GI upset, myalgia, dry mouth/thirst. Rarely
Churg–Strauss syndrome: asthma (± rhinitis/sinusitis) with systemic vasculitis and ↑EØ*.
Monitor: FBC* and for development of vasculitic (purpuric/non-blanching) rash, peripheral neuropathy, ↑respiratory/cardiac symptoms: all signs of possible Churg–Strauss syndrome.

L/R/H = **L**iver, **R**enal and **H**eart failure (full key see p. x)

Dose: 10 mg nocte ($\downarrow$doses if <14 years old[BNF]).

MORNING-AFTER PILL/LEVONELLE-2

High-dose levonorgestrel for emergency conception.
CI/Caution: see BNF/product literature.
SE: N&V, abdominal pain, menstrual Δs, mastalgia, headache, fatigue, dizziness.
Dose: 2×750-μg tablets (1.5 mg total) to be taken together asap (preferably <12 h; but no later than 72 h) post coitus.
NB: $\downarrow$efficacy if taking enzyme-inducing drugs (may need to $\uparrow$dose[BNF]) or if vomiting occurs <3 h after either tablet (must take replacement tablet with antiemetic, preferably domperidone).

MORPHINE

Opioid analgesic.
Use: severe pain (inc post-op), AMI and acute LVF.
CI: acute respiratory depression, $\uparrow$risk of paralytic ileus, acute alcoholism, $\uparrow$ICP/head injury (respiratory depression $\Rightarrow$ CO_2 retention and cerebral vasodilation $\Rightarrow$ $\uparrow$ICP), phaeo.
Caution: $\downarrow$respiratory reserve (esp asthma, COPD), $\downarrow$BP, $\downarrow$T$_4$, $\uparrow$prostate, convulsive disorders, **L** (can $\Rightarrow$ **coma**: avoid using or give minimum dose), **R/P/B/E**.
SE: N&V, **respiratory depression, constipation*** (can $\Rightarrow$ **ileus**), seizures (at $\uparrow$doses), $\downarrow$BP (rarely $\uparrow$BP), sedation, dry mouth, urinary retention, biliary tract spasms, anorexia, mood Δ ($\uparrow$ or $\downarrow$), $\downarrow$libido, **dependence**. Rarely, skin reactions, $\downarrow$Pt.
Interactions: other CNS depressants (use with care).
Dose: 5–15 mg sc/im up to 4-hourly; 2.5–10 mg iv up to 4-hourly (at 2 mg/min). NB: iv doses are generally ¼–⅓ that of im doses. Can $\uparrow$dose and frequency with expert supervision and always adjust dose to response (in chronic pain, can use po as Oramorph, MST or Sevredol; see pp. 141 and 144). *Unless short-term Rx, always consider laxative Px**.

☠If $\downarrow$BMI or elderly, titrate dose up slowly, monitor O_2 sats and have naloxone $\pm$ resuscitation trolley at hand. ☠

MST CONTINUS SR oral morphine available as tablets or solution (*specify which*).
Dose: large range: 5–200 mg bd (adjust to previous daily morphine requirements).

MUPIROCIN/BACTROBAN

Topical antibiotic for bacterial infections (esp nasal MRSA); available as ointment and cream (*specify which*) bd/tds.

Local MRSA eradication protocols often exist; if not, then a sensible regime is to give for 5–10 days and then swab 2 days later, repeating regime if culture still positive.

▼MYCOPHENOLATE MOFETIL (MMF)

Immunosuppressant: ↓s B-/T-cell lymphocytes (and ↓s Ab production by B-cells).
Use: transplant rejection Px, autoimmune diseases, vasculitis.
CI: P/B
Caution: active serious GI diseases, **E**.
Monitor: FBC.
Warn: patient to report unexplained bruises/bleeding/signs of infection. Avoid strong sunlight*.
SE: GI upset, blood disorders (esp ↓NØ, ↓Pt), weakness, tremor, headache, ↑cholesterol, ↑ or ↓K^+. Rarely, hepatotoxicity, skin neoplasms*. *Specialist use only*.

N-ACETYLCYSTEINE see Acetylcysteine; paracetamol antidote.

NALOXONE

Opioid receptor antagonist for opiate reversal if OD or over-Rx.
Dose: 0.8–2.0 mg iv (or sc/im). *Short-acting*: often needs to be repeated every 2–3 min, up to 10 mg total (consider ivi).

NAPROXEN

NSAID (propionic acid derivative): unselective COX inhibitor.
Use: rheumatoid arthritis[1], other musculoskeletal pain[2] (esp post-orthopaedic surgery), acute gout[3], dysmenorrhoea[4].

CI/Caution/SE: as ibuprofen, but more severe SEs.
Dose: 250–500 mg bd[1]; 500 mg initially then 250 mg 6–8-hourly[2,4]; 750 mg initially then 250 mg 8-hourly[3]. Also available with misoprostol as Px against PU (as Napratec).

NARCAN see Naloxone

NICORANDIL

K^+-channel activator with nitrate component ($\therefore \Rightarrow$ venous/arterial dilation).
Use: angina Px/Rx (unresponsive to other Rx).
CI: ↓BP (esp cardiogenic shock), LVF with ↓filling pressures.
Caution: hypovolaemia, acute pulmonary oedema, P/B.
SE: headache (often only initially*), **flushing**, dizziness, weakness, N&V, ↓BP, ↑HR (dose-dependent). Rarely, oral ulcers, myalgia, angioedema, hepatotoxicity.
Dose: 5–30 mg bd (start low, esp if susceptible to headaches*).

NIFEDIPINE

Ca^{++} channel blocker (dihydropyridine): dilates smooth muscle, esp arteries (inc coronaries). Reflex sympathetic drive $\Rightarrow$ ↑HR and ↑contractility $\therefore \Rightarrow$ ↓HF cf other Ca^{++} channel blockers (e.g. verapamil, and to a lesser degree diltiazem), which $\Rightarrow$ ↓HR + ↓contractility. Also has diuretic effects*.
Use: angina Px[1], HTN[2], Raynaud's[3].
CI: cardiogenic shock, severe aortic stenosis, ACS (inc w/in 1 month of MI), porphyria.
Caution: angina or LVF can worsen (consider stopping drug), ↓BP, DM, L (↓dose), R/H/P/B
SE: flushing, headache, ankle oedema, dizziness, ↓**BP**, palpitations, rash/pruritus, GI upset, weakness, myalgia, arthralgia. Rarely, PU, hepatotoxicity and polyuria/nocturia.
Interactions: ↑ fx of digoxin. ↓s fx of quinidine. Ciclosporin and grapefruit juice ↑ fx of nifedipine. Rifampicin, phenytoin and carbamazepine ↓ fx of nifedipine.
Dose: 5–20 mg tds po[3]; use long-acting preparations for HTN/ angina, as normal-release preparations $\Rightarrow$ erratic BP control and

reflex ↑HR, which can worsen IHD (e.g. Adalat LA or Retard and many others with differing fx and doses[BNF]).

NITROFURANTOIN

Antibiotic: 'static' at ↓doses, 'cidal' at ↑doses. Only active in urine (no systemic antibacterial fx).

Use: UTIs.

CI: G6PD deficiency, porphyria, **R** (also ⇒ ↓activity of drug: it needs to be concentrated in urine), **P/B**.

Caution: DM, lung disease, ↓Hb, ↓vitamin B, ↓folate, electrolyte imbalance, susceptibility to peripheral neuropathy, **L/E**.

SE: GI upset, pulmonary reactions (inc effusions, fibrosis), **peripheral neuropathy, hypersensitivity**. Rarely, hepatotoxicity, cholestasis, pancreatitis, arthralgia, alopecia (transient), skin reactions (esp exfoliative dermatitis), blood disorders, BIH.

Dose: 50–100 mg qds po (od nocte if for Px) with food. Not available iv or im.

NB: can ⇒ false positive urinary dipstick for glucose. Can discolour urine.

NORADRENALINE (= NOREPINEPHRINE)

Vasoconstrictor sympathomimetic: stimulates α-receptors ⇒ vasoconstriction.

Use: ↓BP (unresponsive to other Rx)[1], cardiac arrest[2].

CI: ↑BP, **P**.

Caution: thrombosis (coronary/mesenteric/peripheral), Prinzmetal's angina, post-MI, ↑T_4, DM, ↓O_2, ↑CO_2, hypovolaemia (uncorrected), **E**.

SE: can ↓BF to vital organs (esp kidney). Also headache, ↓HR, arrhythmias, peripheral ischaemia. ↑BP if over-Rx.

Dose: 80 μg/ml ivi at 0.16–0.33 ml/min[1] (adjust according to response); 0.5–0.75 ml of 200-μg/ml solution iv stat[2]. (NB: *doses given here are for noradrenaline **acid tartrate**, not **base***).

NUROFEN see Ibuprofen; NB: over-the-counter use can ⇒ poor response to HTN and HF Rx.

NYSTATIN

Polyene antifungal.

Use: candida infections: topically for skin/mucous membranes (esp mouth/vagina); po for GI infections (not absorbed).

SE: GI upset (at ↑doses), skin reactions.

Dose: topically as gel prn; po suspension 500 000–1 000 000 units qds after food (usually for 1 wk) for Rx. 1 000 000 units od for Px.

OLANZAPINE/ZYPREXA

Im

'Atypical' antipsychotic: D_2 and $5HT_2$ (+ mild muscarinic) antagonist.

Use: schizophrenia[NICE], mania.

CI: glaucoma (angle-closure), **B**.

Caution: drugs that ↑QT, dementia, cardiovascular disease (esp if Hx of or ↑risk of CVA/TIA), DM*, ↑prostate, Parkinson's, Hx of epilepsy, blood disorders, paralytic ileus. ↑s fx of alcohol, L/R/H/P/E.

SE: sedation, ↑Wt, ankle oedema, Δ LFTs, postural ↓BP (esp initially ∴ titrate up dose slowly). Rarely, extrapyramidal/ anticholinergic fx (often transient), neuroleptic malignant syndrome. ↑ing reports of hyperglycaemia and ☠**DM/DKA***

Monitor: HbA_{1C} ± CBGs, BP (esp initially).

Interactions: levels ↓d by carbamazepine and smoking.

Dose: 5–20 mg po daily (pref nocte to avoid daytime sedation). Available in 'melt' form for ↓compliance/swallowing (as Velotab) and im for acute sedation (see product literature for dose).

OMEPRAZOLE/LOSEC

PPI: inhibits H^+/K^+ ATPase of parietal cells ⇒ ↓acid secretion.

Use: PU Rx/Px (esp if on NSAIDs), gastro-oesophageal reflux disease (if symptoms severe or complicated by haemorrhage/ ulcers/ stricture)[NICE]. Also used for *H. pylori* eradication and ZE syndrome.

Caution: can mask symptoms of gastric Ca, L/P/B.

SE: GI upset, headache, dizziness, arthralgia, weakness, skin reactions. Rarely, hepatotoxicity, blood disorders, hypersensitivity.

Interactions: ↓ (and ↑) **P450** ∴ many, most importantly ↑s **phenytoin** (& digoxin) levels. ↓s fx of ketoconazole/itraconazole, **W+**.

Dose: 20 mg od po, ↑ing to bd in severe/resistant cases and for
H. pylori eradication (see p. 133); ↓ing to 10 mg od for maintenance
if symptoms are stable. If unable to take po (e.g. perioperatively,
↓GCS, on ITU), give 40 mg iv od (▼) either over 5 min or as ivi.

NB: also specialist use iv for acute bleeds. Usually as 8 mg/h ivi for
72 h if endoscopic evidence of PU (prescribed as divided infusions,
as drug is unstable). Contact pharmacy ± GI team for advice on
indications and exact dosing regimens.

ONDANSETRON

Antiemetic: $5HT_3$ antagonist: acts on central and GI receptors.
Use: N&V, esp if resistant to other Rx or severe postoperative/
chemotherapy-induced.
Caution: GI obstruction, **L** (unless mild), **P/B**.
SE: constipation (or diarrhoea), **headache**, sedation, fatigue, dizziness.
Rarely seizures, chest pain, ↓BP, Δ LFTs, rash, hypersensitivity.
Dose: 8 mg bd po, 16 mg od pr, 8 mg 2–8-hourly iv/im (max
24 mg/day usually (8 mg/day if LF)). Can also give as ivi at 1 mg/h
for max of 24 h. Exact dose and route depends on indication[BNF].

ORAMORPH oral morphine solution for severe pain, esp useful
for prn or breakthrough pain (see p. 144 for use in palliative care).
Dose: 5–10 mg up to 4-hourly (can ↑dose under specialist
supervision).

Solution mostly commonly used is 10 mg/5 ml, but can be
30 mg/5 ml or 100 mg/5 ml.

OTOSPORIN ear drops for otitis externa (esp if fungal infection
suspected): contains antibacterials (neomycin, polymyxin B) and
hydrocortisone.
Dose: 3 drops tds/qds.

OXYBUTYNIN

Anticholinergic (selective M_3 antagonist), antispasmodic (↓s bladder
muscle contractions).

Use: detrusor instability (also neurogenic bladder instability, nocturnal enuresis).
CI: bladder outflow (or GI) obstruction, urinary retention, intestinal atony, severe UC/toxic megacolon, glaucoma, MG, **B**.
Caution: ↑prostate, autonomic neuropathy, hiatus hernia (if reflux), ↑T_4, IHD, arrhythmias, L/R/H/P/E.
SE: antimuscarinic fx (see p. 174), GI upset , palpitations/↑HR, skin reactions – mostly dose-related and reportedly less severe in MR preparations*.
Dose: initially 2.5–5 mg bd po (↑ing if required to max of 5 mg qds) or as Lyrinel XL* 5–30 mg od.

OXYTETRACYCLINE

Tetracycline antibiotic: inhibits ribosomal protein synthesis.
Use: acne vulgaris (and rosacea).
CI/Caution/SE/Interactions: as tetracycline, plus caution in porphyria.
Dose: 250–500 mg qds 1 h before food or on empty stomach.

PAMIDRONATE

Bisphosphonate: ↓s bone turnover.
Use: ↑Ca^{++}[1] (esp metastatic: also ↓s pain), Paget's disease[2].
CI: P/B.
Caution: Hx of thyroid surgery, R/H.
SE: 'flu-like symptoms (inc fever, transient pyrexia), **GI upset** (inc haemorrhage), **dizziness/somnolence** (warn patient common post-dose), ↑ (or ↓) **BP**, seizures, musculoskeletal pain, electrolyte Δs (↓PO_4, ↓ or ↑K^+, ↑Na^+, ↓Mg^{++}), RF, blood disorders.
Dose: 15–90 mg ivi according to indication and Ca^{++} levels[BNF]; *never given regularly for sustained periods.*

PANTOPRAZOLE

PPI; as omeprazole, but ↓interactions.
Dose: 40 mg od po (↓ing to 20 mg maintenance if symptoms allow). If unable to take po (e.g. perioperatively, ↓GCS, on ITU), can give 40 mg iv over ≥2 min or as ivi.

PARACETAMOL

...pyretic (directly influences hypothalamic heat regulation centre),
...ld analgesic (inhibits PGE_2 synthesis in CNS $\Rightarrow$ ↑pain threshold);
...unlike NSAIDs, *has no anti-inflammatory fx*.
Use: pyrexia, mild pain.
Caution: alcohol dependence, L/R.
SE: *all rare*; rash, hypoglycaemia, blood disorders, hepatic (rarely
renal) failure – esp if over-Rx/OD (for Mx, see pp. 193–5).
Interactions: ↑s fx of AZT, **W+**.
Dose: 0.5–1 g qds po/pr prn (for children, see Calpol).

PAROXETINE/SEROXAT

SSRI anti-depressant.
Use: depression, other Ψ disorders (inc anxiety/panic disorder, OCD).
CI/Caution/SE/Interactions: as fluoxetine, but ↓frequency of
agitation/insomnia, although ↑frequency of **antimuscarinic fx**
(see p. 174), **extrapyramidal fx** (see p. 175) and **withdrawal fx***
(dt short $t_{1/2}$: stop slowly).
Dose: 20 mg mane (max 60 mg).

PARVOLEX see Acetylcysteine; antidote for paracetamol poisoning.

PENICILLAMINE

Chelates Cu/Fe $\Rightarrow$ ↑elimination (also acts as DMARD): slow onset
of action (6–12 wks).
Use: Wilson's disease*, Cu/Fe poisoning, rheumatoid arthritis (also
autoimmune hepatitis, cystinuria).
CI: SLE.
Caution: R/P.
SE: can worsen **neurological symptoms***, RF (esp immune
nephritis $\Rightarrow$ proteinuria*: stop drug if severe), **blood disorders** (↓Pt,
↓NØ, agranulocytosis, aplastic ↓Hb), **rashes** (inc SJS, pemphigus),
taste Δs, GI upset (esp nausea, but ↓s if taken with food). Rarely
hepatotoxicity, pancreatitis, autoimmune phenomena:
polymyositis/dermatomyositis, Goodpasture's syndrome, lupus-/
myasthenia-like syndromes.

Monitor: FBC, U&Es, urine dipstick $\pm$ 24-h collection*.
Interactions: antacids and $FeSO_4$ ↓ its absorption. ↓s fx of digoxin.
Dose: 125–2000 mg daily[BNF].

PENICILLIN G see Benzylpenicillin

PENICILLIN V see Phenoxymethylpenicillin

PENTASA see Mesalazine; 'new' aminosalicylate for UC, but with ↓SEs.

PEPPERMINT OIL
Antispasmodic: direct relaxant of GI smooth muscle.
Use: GI muscle spasm, distension (esp IBS).
SE: perianal irritation, indigestion. Rarely rash or other allergy.
Dose: 1–2 capsules tds, before meals and with water.

PERINDOPRIL/COVERSYL
ACE-i.
Use: HTN, HF.
CI/Caution/SE/Interactions: as captopril, plus can ⇒ mood/sleep Δs.
Dose: initially 2 mg od (maintenance 4–8 mg od).

PETHIDINE
Opiate analgesic; less potent than morphine but quicker action
⇒ ↑euphoria ∴ ↑abuse potential ∴ not suitable for chronic use.
Use/CI/Caution/SE: as morphine, but ⇒ ↓constipation and is
contraindicated if severe RF.
Dose: 25–100 mg up to 4-hourly im/sc (can give 2-hourly postoperatively); 25–50 mg up to 4-hourly iv. Available po but used
rarely[BNF].

PHENOBARBITAL (= PHENOBARBITONE)
Barbiturate antiepileptic: potentiates GABA (inhibitory neurotransmitter), antagonises fx of glutamate (excitatory neurotransmitter).

Use: status epilepticus (SEs limit other uses).
Caution: respiratory depression, porphyria, L/R/P/B/E.
SE: respiratory depression, **sedation**, ↓**BP**, ↓HR, ataxia, skin reactions. Rarely, paradoxical excitement (esp in elderly), blood disorders.
Interactions: ↑**P450** ∴ many, most importantly ↓s fx of carbamazepine, Ca++ antagonists, corticosteroids, ciclosporin and OCP. Caution with other sedative drugs (esp benzodiazepines), **W–**.
Dose: total of 10–20 mg/kg as ivi at 50–100 mg/min.

PHENOXYMETHYLPENICILLIN (= PENICILLIN V) as
benzylpenicillin (penicillin G) but active orally: used for ENT/skin infections (esp erisipelas), Px of rheumatic fever/*S. pneumoniae* infections (esp post-splenectomy).
Dose: 0.5–1.0 g qds po (≥30 min before food).

PHENTOLAMINE
α-blocker, short-acting.
Use: HTN 2° to phaeo (esp during surgery).
CI: ↓BP, IHD.
Caution: PU/gastritis, asthma, R/P/B/E.
SE: ↓**BP**, ↑HR, dizziness, weakness, flushing, GI upset, nasal congestion. Rarely, coronary/cerebrovascular occlusion, arrhythmias.
Dose: 2–5 mg iv (repeat if necessary).

PHENYTOIN
Antiepileptic: blocks Na+ channels (stabilises neuronal membranes).
Use: status epilepticus[1], tonic–clonic seizures[2], partial seizures[3].
CI: *if iv* (do not apply if po); sinus ↓HR, Stokes–Adams syndrome, SAN block, 2nd-/3rd-degree HB, porphyria.
Caution: DM, porphyria ↓BP, L/H/P (⇒ cleft lip/palate, congenital heart disease), B.
SE (Acute): *dose-dependent:* **drowsiness** (also confusion/dizziness), **cerebellar fx** (see p. 175), **rash** (common cause of intolerance and rarely ⇒ SJS/TEN), N&V, diplopia, dyskinesia (esp orofacial). *If iv,*

*risk of ↓BP, **arrhythmias*** (esp ↑QT), '**purple glove syndrome**'* (hand damage distal to injection site), CNS/respiratory depression.

SE (Chronic): gum hypertrophy, coarse facies, hirsutism, acne, ↓folate (⇒ megaloblastic ↓Hb), Dupuytren's, peripheral neuropathy, rickets, osteomalacia. Rarely, blood disorders, hepatotoxicity.

Monitor: FBC**, keep serum levels at 10–20 mg/l (narrow therapeutic index). 💀 If iv, closely monitor BP and ECG* (esp QTc) 💀.

Warn: report immediately any rash, mouth ulcers, sore throat, fever, bruising, bleeding.

Interactions: ↑P450 ∴ many, most importantly ↓s fx of OCP, doxycycline, Ca^{++} antagonists, ciclosporin and corticosteriods. Its fx are ↑d by aspirin, amiodarone, metronidazole, chloramphenicol, clarithromycin, isoniazid and sulphonamides. Complex interactions with other antiepileptics[BNF]. **W−** (or rarely **W+**).

Dose: po[2,3], 150–500 mg/day in 1–2 divided doses; **iv**[1], load with 15 mg/kg ivi at max rate of 50 mg/min, then maintenance iv doses of approximately 100 mg tds/qds, adjusting to weight, serum levels and clinical response. If available give iv as *fosphenytoin* (NB: doses differ).

💀 Stop drug if ↓WCC** is severe, worsening or associated with symptoms. 💀

PHOSPHATE ENEMA

Laxative enemas.

Use: severe constipation (unresponsive to other Rx).

CI: acute GI disorders.

Caution: E.

SE: local irritation.

Dose: 1–2 prn.

PHYLLOCONTIN CONTINUS see Aminophylline (MR)

Dose: initially 1 tablet (225 mg) bd po, then ↑ to 2 tablets bd after 1 wk. (Forte tablets of 350 mg used if smoker/other cause of ↓$t_{1/2}$, e.g. interactions with other drugs; see Theophylline.)

PICOLAX see Bowel preparations

Dose: 1 sachet at 8am and 3pm the day before GI surgery or Ix.

▼PIOGLITAZONE/ACTOS

Thiazolidinedione (= glitazone) antidiabetic; see Rosiglitazone.
Use/CI/Caution/SE/Monitor: see Rosiglitazone.
Dose: 15–30 mg od.

PIPERACILLIN

Ureidopenicillin: antipseudomonal.
Use: with tazobactam* (β-lactamase inhibitor), reserved for severe infections.
CI/Caution/SE: see Benzylpenicillin.
Dose: see Tazocin*.

PIRITON see Chlorphenamine; antihistamine for allergies.

PLAVIX see Clopidogrel; anti-Pt agent for Px of IHD (and CVA).

POTASSIUM TABLETS see Kay-cee-L (syrup 1 mmol/ml),
Kloref (effervescent 6.7 mmol/tablet), Sando-K (effervescent
12 mmol/tablet) and Slow-K (MR non-effervescent 8 mmol/tablet,
reserved for when syrup/effervescent preparations are inappropriate;
avoid if ↓swallow).

PRAVASTATIN/LIPOSTAT

HMG-CoA reductase inhibitor.
Use/CI/Caution/SE/Interactions: see Simvastatin (but does not potentiate warfarin).
Dose: 10–40 mg nocte.

PREDNISOLONE

Glucocorticoid (and mild mineralocorticoid activity).
Use: anti-inflammatory (e.g. rheumatoid arthritis, IBD, asthma, eczema), immunosuppression (e.g. transplant rejection Px, acute leukaemias), glucocorticoid replacement (e.g. Addison's disease, hypopituitarism).
CI: systemic infections (w/o antibiotic cover).
Caution/SE/Interactions: see pp. 169–71.

L/R/H = **L**iver, **R**enal and **H**eart failure (full key see p. x)

Warn: carry steroid card (and avoid close contact with people who have chickenpox if patient has never had it).

Dose: usually 2.5–15 mg od po for maintenance. In acute/initial stages, 20–60 mg od often needed (depends on cause and often physician preference), e.g. acute asthma (40 mg od), acute COPD (30 mg od), temporal arteritis (40–60 mg daily). Take with food ($\downarrow Na^+$, $\uparrow K^+$ diet recommended if on long-term Rx). For others causes, consult BNF, pharmacy or local specialist relevant to the disease.

☠ Warn patient not to stop tablets suddenly (*can* $\Rightarrow$ *Addisonian crisis*). Requirements may $\uparrow$ if intercurrent illness/surgery. ☠

PROCHLORPERAZINE/STEMETIL

Antiemetic: DA antagonist (phenothiazine $\therefore$ also antipsychotic, but used rarely for this).

Use: N&V (inc labyrinthine disorders).

CI/Caution/SE: as chlorpromazine, but $\downarrow$sedation and $\uparrow$**extrapyramidal fx**.

Dose: *po*, acutely 20 mg, then 10 mg 2 h later (5–10 mg bd/tds for Px and labyrinthine disorders); *im*, 12.5 mg, then po doses 6 h later; *pr*, 25 mg then po doses 6 h later (5 mg tds pr for migraine). (Buccastem – quick-dissolving buccal 3-mg tablets left under lip, 1–2 bd.)

PROCYCLIDINE

Antimuscarinic: $\downarrow$s cholinergic to dopaminergic ratio in extrapyramidal syndromes $\Rightarrow \downarrow$tremor/rigidity. No fx on bradykinesia (or tardive dyskinesia; may even worsen).

Use: extrapyramidal symptoms (e.g. parkinsonism), esp if drug-induced[1] (e.g. antipsychotics).

CI: urinary retention (if untreated), glaucoma* (angle-closure), GI obstruction.

Caution: cardiovascular disease, $\uparrow$prostate, tardive dyskinesia, **L/R/H/P/B/E**.

SE: antimuscarinic fx (see p. 174), Ψ disturbances, euphoria (can be drug of abuse), glaucoma*.

Dose: 5 mg tds po prn[1] ($\uparrow$ if necessary to max of 10 mg tds);
5–10 mg im/iv if acute dystonia or oculogyric crisis.
NB: do not stop suddenly: can $\Rightarrow$ rebound muscarinic fx.

PROMETHAZINE

Sedating antihistamine.
Use: insomnia (see p. 173).
CI: CNS depression/coma, MAOI w/in 14 days.
Caution: urinary retention, $\uparrow$prostate, glaucoma, epilepsy, IHD,
asthma, porphyria, pyloroduodenal obstruction, **R** ($\downarrow$dose), **L/E/P/B**.
SE: antimuscarinic fx, hangover sedation, headache, psychomotor
impairment.
Dose: 25 mg nocte (can $\uparrow$dose to 50 mg).

PROPRANOLOL

β-blocker (nonselective): $\beta_1 \Rightarrow \downarrow$HR and $\downarrow$contractility, $\beta_2 \Rightarrow$
vasodilation (and bronchoconstriction and glucose release from
liver). Also blocks fx of catecholamines, $\downarrow$s renin production, slows
SAN/AVN conduction.
Use: HTN[1], IHD (angina Rx[2], MI Px[3]), portal HTN[4] (*may worsen
liver function*), essential tremor[5], Px of migraine[6], anxiety[7], $\uparrow$T$_4$
(symptom relief[8], thyroid storm[9]), arrhythmias[8] (inc severe[9]).
CI: asthma/Hx of bronchospasm, peripheral arterial disease
(if severe), Prinzmetal's angina, severe $\downarrow$HR or $\downarrow$BP, SSS, 2nd-/3rd-
degree HB, cardiogenic shock, metabolic acidosis, phaeo (unless
used specifically with α-blockers), **H** (if uncontrolled).
Caution: COPD, 1st-degree HB, DM*, MG, Hx of hypersensitivity
(may $\uparrow$ to *all* allergens), **L/R/P/B**.
SE: $\downarrow$HR, $\downarrow$BP, HF, peripheral vasoconstriction ($\Rightarrow$ cold
extremities, worsening of claudication/Raynaud's), **fatigue,
depression, sleep disturbance** (inc nightmares), hyperglycaemia
(and $\downarrow$**sympathetic response to *hypo*glycaemia***), GI upset. Rarely,
conduction/blood disorders.
Interactions: 🐍**verapamil and diltiazem** $\Rightarrow$ **risk of HB and**
$\downarrow$**HR** 💀. Antihypertensive fx $\downarrow$d by NSAIDs (Mild **W+**).

Dose: 80–160 mg bd po[1]; 40–120 mg bd po[2]; 40 mg qds for 2–3 days, then 80 mg bd po[3] (start 5–21 days post-MI); 40 mg bd po[4] (↑dose if necessary); 40 mg bd/tds po[5,6]; 40 mg od po[7] (↑dose to tds if necessary); 10–40 mg tds/qds[8]; 1 mg iv over 1 min[9] (repeating every 2 min if required, to max of 10 mg).

NB: ↓po dose in LF and ↓initial dose in RF. Withdraw slowly (esp in angina; as can ⇒ rebound worsening of symptoms).

PROPYLTHIOURACIL

Thionamide anti-thyroid: peroxidase inhibitor – stops I^- conversion to I_2 and ∴ ↓s $T_{3/4}$ production (as carbimazole), but also ↓s peripheral T_4 to T_3 conversion and possible immunosuppressant fx.

Use: ↑T_4 (2nd-line in the UK; if carbimazole not tolerated).
Caution: L/R, P/B (can cause fetal/neonatal goitre/↓T_4 ∴ use min dose and monitor neonatal development closely; 'block and-replace' regimen ∴ not suitable as high doses used).
SE: blood disorders (esp **agranulocytosis**; stop drug if occurs), **skin reactions** (esp urticaria, rarely cutaneous vasculitis/lupus), fever. Rarely hepatotoxicity, nephritis.
Warn: patient to seek medical advice if symptoms of infection (esp sore throat).
Monitor: FBC, clotting (mild **W+**).
Dose: 200–400 mg od po until euthyroid, then ↓ to 50–150 mg od.

PROSCAR see Finasteride; antiandrogen for BPH (and baldness).

PROTAMINE (SULPHATE)

Protein (basic) that binds heparin (acidic).
Use: reversal of heparin following over-Rx/OD or after temporary anticoagulation for extracorporeal circuits (e.g. cardiopulmonary bypass, haemodialysis).
SE: ↓**BP**, ↓HR, N&V, flushing, dyspnoea. Rarely pulmonary oedema, hypertension, **hypersensitivity reactions**.

Dose: 1 mg per 80–100 units of heparin to be reversed as ivi over 10 min. NB: $t_{1/2}$ of iv heparin is short; ↓doses of protamine if giving >15 mins after last iv heparin administration.

Max total dose 50 mg: 💀*high doses can ⇒ anticoagulant fx!*💀

PROZAC see Fluoxetine; SSRI antidepressant.

PULMICORT see Budesonide; inh steroid for asthma. 50, 100, 200 or 400 µg/puff.

PYRAZINAMIDE
Antibiotic: 'cidal' only against intracellular and dividing bacteria (e.g. TB). Good CSF penetration*.
Use: TB Rx (for initial phase, see p. 131), TB meningitis*.
CI: porphyria, **L**.
Caution: DM, gout (avoid in acute attacks), **P**.
SE: hepatotoxicity**, ↑**urate**, GI upset (inc N&V), dysuria, interstitial nephritis, arthralgia/myalgia, sideroblastic ↓Hb, ↓Pt, rash (and photosensitivity).
Monitor: LFTs**.
Dose: up to 2 g daily – exact dose varies according to Wt and whether Rx is 'supervised' or not[BNF].

PYRIDOSTIGMINE
Anticholinesterase: inhibits cholinesterase at neuromuscular junction ⇒ ↑ACh ⇒ ↑neuromuscular transmission.
Use: myasthenia gravis.
CI: GI/urinary obstruction.
Caution: asthma, recent MI, ↓HR, arrhythmias, vagotonia, ↑T_4, PU, epilepsy, parkinsonism, **R/P/B**.
SE: cholinergic fx (see p. 174) – esp if xs Rx/OD, where ↓BP, bronchoconstriction and (confusingly) weakness can also occur (= cholinergic crisis*); ↑**secretions** (sweat/saliva/tears) and miosis are good clues** of xs ACh.
Interactions: fx ↓d by aminoglycosides (e.g. gentamicin), clindamycin, lithium, quinidine, chloroquine, propranolol and procainamide. It ↑s fx of suxamethonium.

L/R/H = **L**iver, **R**enal and **H**eart failure (full key see p. x)

Dose: 300–1200 mg daily po according to response (usually in 2–4 doses of 30–120 mg, e.g. 60 mg qds).

☠ ↑ing weakness can be due to *cholinergic crisis** as well as MG exacerbation; if unsure which is responsible**, get senior help (esp if ↓respiratory function) before giving Rx, as the wrong choice can be fatal! ☠

QUININE
Antimalarial: kills bloodborne schizonts.
Use: malaria Rx[1] (esp falciparum), (nocturnal) leg cramps[2].
CI: optic neuritis, haemoglobinuria, MG*.
Caution: heart conduction dfx (inc AF, HB), G6PD deficiency, P.
SE: visual Δs (inc temporary blindness, esp in OD), **tinnitus** (and vertigo/deafness), **GI upset**, **headache**, **rash/flushing**, **hypersensitivity**, confusion, hypoglycaemia**. Rarely blood disorders, ARF, cardiovascular fx (can ⇒ severe ↓BP in OD).
Monitor: blood glucose** (if given iv).
Interactions: ↑s fx of flecainide and digoxin. ↑s risk of arrhythmias with antipsychotics and amiodarone. Antagonises anticholinesterases.*
Dose: 200–300 mg nocte po[2]. *For malaria Rx, see pp. 133–4.*

RAMIPRIL/TRITACE
ACE-i.
Use: HTN[1], HF[2], Px post-MI[3]. Also Px of cardiovascular disease (if age >55 years and at risk)[4].
CI/Caution/SE/Interactions: as captopril.
Dose: initially 1.25 mg od (↑ing slowly to max of 10 mg od)[1,2]; initially 2.5 mg bd then ↑ to 5.0 mg bd after 2 days[3] (start 3–10 days post-MI); initially 2.5 mg od (↑ing to 10 mg)[4].

RANITIDINE/ZANTAC
H_2 antagonist ⇒ ↓parietal cell H^+ secretion.
Use: PU (Px if on longterm high dose NSAIDs[1], chronic Rx[2], acute Rx[3]), *H. pylori* eradication, reflux oesophagitis.
Caution: porphyria, L/R/P/B. ☠ *May mask symptoms of gastric cancer.* ☠

SE: *all rare:* GI upset (esp diarrhoea), dizziness, confusion, fatigue, blurred vision, headache, Δ LFTs (rarely hepatitis), rash. Very rarely arrhythmias (esp if given iv), hypersensitivity, blood disorders.

Interactions: minimal cf cimetidine.

Dose: initially 150 mg bd po (or 300 mg nocte)[1,2], ↑ing to 600 mg/day if necessary but try to ↓ to 150 mg nocte for maintenance; 50 mg tds/qds iv[3] (or im/ivi[BNF]).

REOPRO see Abciximab

RETEPLASE (= r-PA)

Recombinant plasminogen activator: thrombolytic.

Use/CI/Caution/SE: see Alteplase and pp. 161–3 but only for Rx of AMI.

Dose: 10 units iv over 2 min, then repeat after 30 min. Concurrent unfractionated iv heparin needed for 48 h; see p. 163.

RIFABUTIN

New rifamycin antibiotic; see Rifampicin.

Use: TB: Rx of pulmonary TB[1] and non-tuberculous mycobacterial disease.[2] Also Px of *M. avium*[3] (if HIV with ↓CD4).

CI/Caution/SE/Interations: see Rifampicin.

Dose: 150–450 mg od[1]; 450–600 mg od[2]; 300 mg od[3].

RIFAMPICIN

Rifamycin antibiotic: 'cidal' ⇒ ↓RNA synthesis.

Use: TB Rx, *N. meningitides* (meningococcal)/*H. influenzae* (type b) meningitis Px. Rarely for *Legionella*/*Brucella*/*Staphylococcus* infections.

CI: jaundice.

Caution: porphyria, L/R/P/B.

SE: hepatotoxicity, GI upset (inc AAC), headache, fever, 'flu-like symptoms, orange/red body secretions, SOB, blood disorders, skin reactions, shock, ARF.

Warn: of symptoms/signs of liver disease; report jaundice/persistent N&V/malaise immediately.

Monitor: LFTs, FBC (and U&Es if dose >600 mg/day).

Interactions: ↑**P450** ∴ many; most importantly ↓**s fx of OCP***, carbamazepine, phenytoin, sulphonylureas, corticosteroids and Ca^{++} antagonists; **W–**.

Dose: for TB Rx, see p. 131; for other indications see BNF. (NB: well absorbed po; give iv *only* if ↓swallow.)

Other contraception* needed during Rx.

RIFATER combination preparation of rifampicin, isoniazid and pyrazinamide for 1st 2 months of TB Rx (⇒ ↓bacterial load/ infectiousness until sensitivities known); see p. 131.

RISEDRONATE

Bisphosphonate. ↓s bone turnover.

Use: osteoporosis (Px^1/Rx^2, esp if postmenopausal or steroid-induced), Paget's disease[3].

CI: ↓Ca^{++}, **P/B**.

Caution: delayed GI transit/emptying (esp oesophageal abnormalities), **R**.

SE: GI upset, bone/joint/muscle pain, headache, rash, HTN. Rarely chest pain, oedema, ↓Wt, apnoea, bronchitis, sinusitis, glossitis, nocturia, infections (esp UTIs), amblyopia, iritis, dry eyes/ corneal lesions, tinnitus.

Warn: take with full glass of water on an empty stomach ≥30 min before, and stay upright until, breakfast*.

Interactions: Ca^{++}-containing products (ine milk) and antacids (⇒ ↓absorption) ∴ separate doses as much as possible from risedronate.

Dose: 5 mg od[1,2] (or 1 × 35-mg tablet/week as ▼Actonel once a week[2]).

RISPERIDONE/RISPERDAL

'Atypical' antipsychotic: similar to olanzapine (⇒ ↓extrapyramidal fx cf 'typical' antipsychotics, esp tardive dyskinesia)

Use/CI/Caution/SE/Interactions: Similar to olanzapine but ⇒ ↓sedation, ↑hypotension (esp initially: ↑dose slowly) and ↑prolactin.

Dose: 0.5 mg–8 mg bd po. Also available as liquid or quick dissolving 1 mg/2 mg tablets ("Quicklets") and as long acting im 2 weekly injections ("Consta" ▼) for ↑compliance.

RIVASTIGMINE/EXELON

Acetylcholinesterase inhibitor that acts centrally (crosses BBB): replenishes ACh, which is ↓d in certain dementias.

Use: Alzheimer's disease[NICE].

CI: B.

Caution: conduction defects (esp SSS), PU susceptibility, COPD/asthma, bladder outflow obstruction, **L/R/P**.

SE: cholinergic fx (see p. 174), **GI upset, headache, dizziness,** behavioural/Ψ reactions. Rarely GI haemorrhage, ↓HR, AV block, angina, seizures, rash.

Interactions: P450 ∴ many – see BNF/product literature.

Dose: 1.5 mg bd initially (↑d to 3–6 mg bd: specialist review needed for clinical response and tolerance).

ROFECOXIB/VIOXX

NSAID: selective COX2 inhibitor.

Use/CI/Caution/SE/Interactions: as celecoxib, plus used in acute pain other than arthritis and caution in IHD.

Monitor: LFTs (stop drug if persistently raised).

Dose: 12.5–50 mg od.

▼ROSIGLITAZONE/AVANDIA

Thiazolidinedione (= glitazone) antidiabetic: ↓s peripheral insulin resistance (and, to lesser extent, hepatic gluconeogenesis).

Use: type 2 DM, currently only recommended in combination with sulphonylurea or (preferably – esp if obese) metformin[NICE].

CI: insulin use (↑risk of HF), **H** (inc Hx of), **L/P/B**.

Caution: cardiovascular disease, **R**.

SE: oedema (esp if HTN/CCF), ↓**Hb**, ↑**Wt**, GI upset (esp diarrhoea), headache, hypoglycaemia (if also taking sulphonylureas), rarely **hepatotoxicity**.

Monitor: LFTs. ☠*Discontinue if jaundice develops.*☠
Dose: 4 mg od (can ↑dose to max 8 mg/day if given with metformin).

(r)tPA = (Recombinant) tissue-type plasminogen activator; see Alteplase

SALBUTAMOL

β_2 agonist, short-acting: dilates bronchial smooth muscle (and endometrium: also β_2 receptors), inhibits mast-cell mediator release.
Use: chronic[1] and acute[2] asthma. Rarely ↑K^+ (nebs prn), premature labour (iv).
Caution: cardiovascular disease (esp arrhythmias*, HTN), DM (can ⇒ DKA, esp if iv ∴ monitor GBGs), ↑T_4, **P/B**.
SE: *neurological:* **fine tremor**, headache, nervousness, sleep/behavioural Δs (esp in children); *CVS:* ↑**HR**, palpitations/arrhythmias (esp if iv), ↑QT interval*; *other:* ↓K^+, muscle cramps. Rarely hypersensitivity, **paradoxical bronchospasm**.
Interactions: theophyllines, diuretics and corticosteroids ↑risk of ↓K^+.
Dose: 100–400 μg prn inh[1] (aerosol or powder); 2.5–5 mg qds–4-hourly neb[2]. If life-threatening (see pp. 182–3), can ↑nebs up to every 15 min or give as ivi (initially 5 μg/min, then up to 20 μg/min according to response).

SALMETEROL/SEREVENT

Bronchodilator: long-acting β_2 agonist (LABA).
Use: 1st choice add-on for asthma Rx (on top of short-acting β_2 agonist and inh steroids; see BTS guidelines, p. 139). *Not for acute Rx!*
Caution/SE/Interactions: as salbutamol.
Dose: 50–100 μg bd inh.

SALOFALK see Mesalazine; 'new' aminosalicylate for UC (↓SEs).

SANDO-K
Effervescent oral KCl (12 mmol K^+/tablet).
Use: $\downarrow K^+$.
CI: R (if severe).
Caution: GI ulcer/stricture, hiatus hernia ($\downarrow$dose in RF/elderly, $\uparrow$ if established $\downarrow K^+$).
SE: N&V, GI ulceration.
Dose: according to serum K^+: average 2–4 tablets/day if normal diet.

SENNA/SENOKOT
Stimulant laxative.
Use: constipation.
CI: GI obstruction.
SE: GI cramps (if chronic use risk of atonic non-functioning colon and $\downarrow K^+$).
Dose: 2 tablets nocte.

SEPTRIN see Co-trimoxazole (sulfamethoxazole + trimethoprim).

SERC see Betahistine; histamine analogue for vestibular disorders.

SEROXAT see Paroxetine; SSRI antidepressant.

SERETIDE combination asthma inhaler with possible synergistic action: long-acting β_2 agonist (LABA); salmeterol 50 µg (Accuhaler) or 25 µg (Evohaler) + fluticasone (steroid) in varying quantities (50, 100, 125, 250 or 500 µg/puff).

SERTRALINE/LUSTRAL
SSRI antidepressant.
Use: depression, OCD.
CI/Caution/SE/Interactions: as fluoxetine, but $\downarrow$incidence of agitation/insomnia.
Dose: 50–100 mg od (max daily dose 200 mg; if >100 mg/day, must be divided into at least 2 doses).

▼SEVELAMER/RENAGEL

PO_4-binding agent; contains no aluminium/Ca^{++} ∴ no risk of ↑ing their levels (which can occur with other drugs, esp if on dialysis). Also ↓s cholesterol.

Use: ↑PO_4 (if on dialysis).

CI: GI obstruction.

Caution: GI disorders, **P/B**.

SE: GI upset, ↓ (or ↑) BP, headache.

Dose: initially 800–1612 mg tds po (as 403-mg capsules or 800-mg tablets), then adjust according to response.

SEVREDOL oral m orphine tablets[1] or solution[2].
Dose: 10–50 mg[1] or 10–20 mg[2] up to 4-hourly.

SILDENAFIL/VIAGRA

Phosphodiesterase type 5 inhibitor: ↑s local fx of NO (⇒ ↑smooth-muscle relaxation ∴ ↑BF into corpus cavernosum).

Use: erectile dysfunction.

CI: recent MI/CVA, ↓BP, unstable angina, hereditary degenerative retinal disorders.

Caution: cardiovascular disease, bleeding disorders (inc active PU), anatomical deformation of penis, predisposition to prolonged erection (e.g. multiple myeloma/leukaemias/sickle cell disease), **L/R/H**.

SE: headache, flushing, GI upset, dizziness, visual disturbances, nasal congestion, hypersensitivity reactions. Rarely, serious cardiovascular events.

Interactions: ⚠ *Nitrates (e.g. GTN/ISMN/ISDN/nicorandil) can ↓↓BP ∴ never give together.* ⚠ Antivirals (esp ritonavir) ↑ its levels.

Dose: 25–100 mg 1 h before intercourse.

SIMVASTATIN/ZOCOR

HMG-CoA reductase inhibitor: ⇒ ↓cholesterol (↓s synthesis), ↓LDL (↑s uptake), mildly ↓s TG.

Use: ↑cholesterol, Px of atherosclerotic disease: IHD (inc 1° prevention), CVA, PVD.

CI: porphyria, **L/P/B**.

Caution: ↓T_4, alcohol abuse, Hx of liver disease, **R** (if severe).

SE: hepatitis and **myositis*** (both rare but important), headache, GI upset, rash, hypersensitivity.

Monitor: LFTs (and CK if symptoms develop*).

Interactions: myositis* ↑d by fibrates, nicotinic acid, clarithromycin, erythromycin, itraconazole, ketoconazole, ciclosporin and protease inhibitors **W+**.

Dose: 10–80 mg nocte (usually start at 20 mg).

☠ Myositis* can rarely ⇒ **rhabdomyolysis**, esp if ↓T_4, RF or taking certain drugs: see interactions. ☠

SINEMET see Co-careldopa; L-dopa + peripheral dopa-decarboxylase inhibitor.

SLOW-K

Slow-release (non-effervescent) oral KCl (8 mmol K^+/tablet).

Use: ↓K^+ *where liquid/effervescent tablets inappropriate.*

CI/Caution/SE: as Sando-K, plus caution if ↓swallow.

Dose: according to serum K^+: average 3–6 tablets/day.

SODIUM BICARBONATE iv

Alkalinising agent.

Use: metabolic acidosis (esp if RF, DKA or prolonged cardiac arrest), certain drug ODs (esp aspirin), rarely for severe ↑K^+.

SE: paradoxical intracellular acidosis, ↓s O_2 delivery (O_2 saturation curve shift), ↑Na^+, ↑serum osmolality.

Dose: *iv:* available in 1.26%, 4.2% and 8.4% solutions; *specialist use only* – get senior help if considering use.

☠ Toxic if extravasation when given iv (⇒ tissue necrosis). ☠

SODIUM VALPROATE see Valproate

SOTALOL

β-blocker: nonselective (class II antiarrhythmic agent plus additional class III activity).

Use: Px of SVT (esp of paroxysmal AF), **Rx of VT** (if life-threatening/symptomatic, esp non-sustained or spontaneous sustained dt IHD or cardiomyopathy), Px of ventricular ectopics.
CI: as propranolol, plus ↑QT syndromes, torsades de pointes, **R** (↓dose if only renal impairment).
Caution: as propranolol, plus electrolyte Δs (⇒ ↑risk of arrhythmias, esp if ↓K+/↓Mg++; ∴ beware if severe diarrhoea).
SE: as propranolol, plus arrhythmias (can ⇒ ↑QT ± **torsades de pointes***, esp in females).
Interactions: 💀*Verapamil and diltiazem ⇒ risk of ↓HR and HB.* 💀 Amiodarone, TCAs and antipsychotics ⇒ ↑**risk arrhythmias***.
Dose: 40–160 mg bd po; 20–120 mg iv over 10 min (repeat 6-hourly if necessary).
Give under specialist supervision and with ECG monitoring.

▼SPIRIVA see Tiotropium; new inhaled muscarinic antagonist.

SPIRONOLACTONE

K+-sparing diuretic: aldosterone antagonist at distal tubule (also potentiates loop and thiazide diuretics).
Use: ascites (esp 2° to cirrhosis or malignancy), oedema, HF (adjunct to ACE-i and/or another diuretic), nephrotic syndrome, 1° aldosteronism.
CI: ↑K+, ↓Na+, Addison's, **P/B**.
Caution: porphyria, **L/R/E**.
SE: ↑K+, **gynaecomastia**, GI upset (inc N&V), impotence, ↓BP, ↑Na+, rash, confusion, headache, hepatotoxicity, blood disorders.
Interactions: ↑s digoxin and lithium levels. ↑s risk of RF with NSAIDs (which also antagonise its diuretic fx).
Dose: 100–400 mg/day po (25 mg od in HF).
💀Beware if on other drugs that ↑K+, e.g. amiloride, triamterene, ACE-i, angiotensin II antagonists and ciclosporin. Do not give with oral K+ supplements inc dietary salt substitutes. 💀

STEMETIL see Prochlorperazine; DA antagonist antiemetic.

STREPTOKINASE

Thrombolytic agent: ↑s plasminogen conversion to plasmin
⇒ ↑fibrin breakdown.

Use: AMI, TE of arteries (inc PE, central retinal artery) or veins
(DVT, central retinal vein).

CI/Caution/SE: see pp. 161–3.

Dose: *MI:* 1.5 million units ivi over 60 min; *other indications:*
250 000 units ivi over 30 min, then 100 000 units ivi every hour for
up to 12–72 h (see product literature).

STREPTOMYCIN

Aminoglycoside antibiotic.

Use: TB (if isoniazid resistance established before Rx); see p. 131.

CI/Caution/SE: see Gentamicin.

SULFAMETHOXAZOLE + TRIMETHOPRIM

see Co-trimoxazole (Septrin)

SULFASALAZINE

Aminosalicylate: combination of 5-aminosalicylic acid (5-ASA) and
sulfapyridine (a sulphonamide).

Use: rheumatoid arthritis[1]. Also UC[2] (inc maintenance of remission)
and active Crohn's disease[2], but not 1st-line, as newer drugs
(e.g. mesalazine) have fewer sulphonamide SEs; still used in those
already well-controlled with this drug and with no SEs or if joint
manifestations.

CI: sulphonamide or salicylate hypersensitivity, **R** (caution if mild).

Caution: slow acetylators, Hx of any allergy, porphyria, G6PD
deficiency, **L/P/B**.

SE: GI upset (esp ↓appetite, ↓Wt), **hepatotoxicity, blood
disorders, hypersensitivity** (inc severe skin reactions), seizures,
lupus.

Monitor: LFTs, U&Es, FBC.

Dose: 500 mg/day ↑ing to max 3 g/day[1]; 1–2 g qds po for acute
attacks[2], ↓ing to maintenance of 500 mg qds – can also give 0.5–1.0 g
pr bd after motion (as supps) ± po Rx or 3 g pr nocte (as enema).

SYMBICORT combination asthma inhaler: each puff contains long-acting β_2 agonist (LABA) formoterol 4.5 µg + steroid budesonide 80 µg (as 100/6 preparation), 160 µg (as 200/6 preparation) or 320 µg (as 400/12 preparation).

SYNACTHEN = SYNthetic ACTH (adrenocorticotrophic hormone)
Use: Dx of Addison's disease; in 'short' test will find ↓plasma cortisol 0, 30 and 60 mins after 250 µg iv/im dose.
CI/Caution/SE: as steroids (pp. 169–70); can also ⇒ anaphylaxis.

TACROLIMUS (= FK 506)
Immunosuppressant (calcineurin inhibitor): ↓s IL-2-mediated LØ proliferation.
Use: Px of transplant rejection (esp renal).
CI: macrolide hypersensitivity, **P/B**.
Caution/SE: as ciclosporin, but ⇒ ↑neuro-/nephrotoxicity (although ⇒ ↓hypertrichosis/hirsutism); also **diabetogenic** and rarely ⇒ cardiomyopathy.
Interactions: levels ↑d by clarithromycin/erythromycin, chloramphenicol, antifungals, ritonavir/nelfinavir, nifedipine and diltiazem. Levels ↓d by rifampicin. Nephrotoxicity ↑d by NSAIDs and amphotericin. Avoid with other drugs that can ↑K+.
Dose: specialist use[BNF].
Interactions important: ↑levels ⇒ toxicity; ↓levels may ⇒ rejection.

TAMOXIFEN
Oestrogen receptor antagonist.
Use: oestrogen receptor-positive Ca breast[1] (as adjuvant Rx: ⇒ ↑survival, delays metastasis), anovulatory infertility[2].
CI: P (*exclude before starting Rx*).
Caution: ↑risk of TE (if taking cytotoxics), porphyria, **B**.
SE: hot flushes, GI upset, menstrual/endometrial Δs (☠inc Ca: if Δ vaginal bleeding/discharge or pelvic pain/pressure ⇒ urgent Ix☠). Also fluid retention, exac of bony metastases pain. Many other gynaecological/blood/skin/metabolic Δs (esp lipids, LFTs).

Interactions: W+.
Dose: 20 mg od po[1].

TAMSULOSIN/FLOMAX MR*

α_1 blocker $\Rightarrow$ internal urethral sphincter relaxation ($\therefore \Rightarrow \uparrow$bladder outflow) and systemic vasodilation.
Use: BPH.
CI/Caution/SE: as Doxazosin plus **L** (if severe).
Dose: 400 µg mane (after food). Available in MR preparation*.

TAZOCIN combination of piperacillin (antipseudomonal penicillin) + tazobactam (β-lactamase inhibitor).
Use: severe infections/sepsis (mostly in ITU setting or if resistant to other antibiotics).
CI/Caution/SE: as Benzylpenicillin plus **R**.
Dose: 2.25–4.5 g tds/qds iv.

TEGRETOL see Carbamazepine; antiepileptic.

TEICOPLANIN

Glycopeptide antibiotic.
Use: serious Gram-positive infections (mostly reserved for MRSA).
Caution: vancomycin sensitivity, **R/P/B**.
SE: GI upset, **hypersensitivity/skin reactions**, **blood disorders**, nephrotoxicity, ototoxicity (but less than vancomycin), ΔLFTs, local reactions at injection site.
Monitor: U&Es, LFTs, FBC, auditory function (esp if chronic Rx or on other ototoxic/nephrotoxic drugs, e.g. gentamicin).
Dose: single loading dose of 400 mg im/iv, then $\downarrow$ to 200 mg od 24 h later (if severe infection continue at 400 mg 12-hourly for 2 more doses before changing to 200 mg od; if life threatening then change to 400 mg od). $\uparrow$dose if weight >85 kg, severe burns or endocarditis and $\downarrow$dose if RF; see product literature.

TELMISARTAN/MICARDIS

Angiotensin II antagonist.
Use: HTN.

CI: biliary obstruction, **L/R** (if either severe). **P/B**.
Caution/SE/Interactions: see Losartan.
Dose: 40–80 mg od.

TEMAZEPAM

Benzodiazepine, short-acting.
Use: insomnia.
CI/Caution/SE/Interactions: see Diazepam.
Dose: 10 mg nocte (can ↑dose if tolerant to benzodiazepines, but beware respiratory depression). *Dependency common:* max 4-wk Rx.

TENECTEPLASE (= TNK-tPA)/METALYSE

New recombinant thrombolytic agent; advantage of being given as single bolus.
Use: AMI.
CI/Caution/SE: see pp. 161–3.
Dose: iv bolus over 10 s according to weight: ≥90 kg, 50 mg; 80–89 kg, 45 mg; 70–79 kg, 40 mg; 60–69 kg, 35 mg; <60 kg, 30 mg. Concurrent unfractionated iv heparin needed for 24–48 h; see p. 163.

TERAZOSIN/HYTRIN

α_1 blocker ⇒ internal urethral sphincter relaxation (∴ ⇒ ↑bladder outflow) and systemic vasodilation.
Use: BPH (and rarely HTN).
Caution: Hx of micturition syncope or postural ↓BP, P/B.
SE: see Doxazosin.
Dose: initially 1 mg nocte, ↑ing as necessary (max 20 mg/day). '1st-dose collapse' common.

TERBINAFINE/LAMISIL

Antifungal.
Use: ringworm[1] (tinea spp), dermatophyte nail infections[2].
Caution: psoriasis (may worsen), L/R/P/B.
SE: headache, GI upset, mild rash, joint/muscle pains.
Rarely neuro-Ψ disturbances, blood disorders, hepatic

dysfunction, serious skin reactions (stop drug if progressive rash).
Dose: 250 mg od po for 2–6 wks[1] or 6 wks – 3 months[2].

TERBUTALINE

Inhaled β_2 agonist similar to salbutamol.
Dose: 250–500 μg od–qds inh (powder or aerosol); 5–10 mg up to qds neb. Can also give po/sc/im/iv[BNF].

TETRACYCLINE

Tetracycline antibiotic: inhibits ribosomal (30S subunit) protein synthesis.
Use: acne vulgaris (or rosacea), genital/tropical infections (doxycycline often preferred).
CI: age <12 years (**stains/deforms teeth**), **R/P/B**.
Caution: may worsen MG or SLE, L.
SE: GI upset (rarely AAC), oesophageal irritation, headache, dysphagia. Rarely hepatotoxicity, blood disorders, photosensitivity, hypersensitivity, visual Δs (rarely 2° to BIH; stop drug if suspected).
Interactions: ↓absorption with milk (do not drink 1 h before or 2 h after drug), antacids and Fe/Al/Ca/Mg/Zn salts. ↓s fx of OCP (small risk). Mild **W+**.
Dose: 250 mg qds po (max 500 mg tds/qds).
NB: take >30 min before food.

THEOPHYLLINE

Methylxanthine bronchodilator. *Theories of action:* 1. ↑s intracellular cAMP; 2. adenosine antagonist; 3. ↓s diaphragm fatigue. NB: additive fx with β_2 agonists (but with ↑risk of SEs, esp ↓K^+).
Use: severe asthma/COPD: acute (iv as aminophylline; see pp. 181–3) or chronic (po; see p. 139 for BTS asthma guidelines).
Caution: cardiac disease (risk of arrhythmias*), epilepsy, ↑T_4, PU, HTN, fever, porphyria, **L/P/B/E**.
SE: (tachy)**arrhythmias***, seizures (esp if given rapidly iv), **GI upset** (esp **nausea**), CNS stimulation (restlessness, insomnia), headache, ↓K^+.

Monitor: serum levels, as narrow therapeutic window (10–20 mg/l); toxic fx can occur even in this range.

Interactions: P450 ($\Rightarrow$ very variable $t_{1/2}$): **levels $\uparrow$d** in HF/liver disease/viral infections/elderly, and if taking cimetidine/ciprofloxacin/erythromycin/clarithromycin/fluconazole/ketoconazole/OCP/diltiazem/verapamil. **Levels $\downarrow$d** in smokers/chronic alcohol abuse, and if taking phenytoin/carbamazepine/phenobarbital/rifampicin/ritonavir.

Dose: 125–250 mg tds/qds po (MR preparations often preferred, as $\downarrow$SE; 4 brands available, all different doses[BNF]). NB: available iv as aminophylline.

THIAMINE (= vitamin B$_1$)
Use: replacement for nutritional deficiencies (esp in alcoholism).
Dose: 100 mg tds po in severe deficiency (25 mg od if mild/chronic). For iv preparations, see Pabrinex and pp. 147–8 for Mx of acute alcohol withdrawal.

THYROXINE (= LEVOTHYROXINE)
Synthetic T$_4$ (NB: thyroxine often now called 'levothyroxine').
Use: $\downarrow$T$_4$ Rx (for maintenance); NB: acutely, liothyronine (T$_3$) often needed – see p. 189.
CI: $\uparrow$T$_4$.
Caution: panhypopituitarism/other predisposition to adrenal insufficiency (*corticosteroids needed first*), chronic $\downarrow$T$_4$, cardiovascular disorders*, DI, DM** , P/B/E. xs dose can $\Rightarrow$ osteoporosis.
SE: features of $\uparrow$T$_4$ (should be minimal unless xs Rx): D&V, tremors, restlessness, headache, flushing, sweating, heat intolerance, angina, arrhythmias, palpitations, $\uparrow$HR, muscle cramps/weakness, $\downarrow$Wt.
Interactions: can Δ digoxin and antidiabetic** requirements, $\uparrow$fx TCAS. **W+.**
Dose: 25–200 µg mane (titrate up slowly, esp if elderly/HTN/IHD*).

TINZAPARIN/INNOHEP
Low-molecular-weight heparin.

Use: DVT/PE Rx[1] and Px[2] (inc preoperative). Not licensed for MI/unstable angina (unlike other LMWHs).
CI/Caution/SE: see Heparin. Also caution in asthma (⇒ ↑hypersensitivity reactions.)
Dose: (all sc) 175 units/kg od[1]; 50 units/kg od[2] (3500 units od if low risk).

Monitoring (via anti Xa) needed if RF (i.e. creatinine > 150), pregnancy, Wt >100 kg or <45 kg; see p. 158.

▼TIOTROPIUM/SPIRIVA

New long-acting inh muscarinic antagonist for asthma; similar to ipratropium, but only for chronic use and caution in RF.
Dose: 18 µg od inh.

TIROFIBAN/AGGRASTAT

Anti-Pt agent: glycoprotein IIb/IIIa receptor inhibitor ∴ stops binding of fibrinogen and inhibits Pt aggregation.
Use: Px of MI in unstable angina/NSTEMI (*if last episode of chest pain <12 h*), esp if high risk and awaiting PCI[NICE] (see p. 180).
CI: abnormal bleeding or CVA w/in 30 days, bleeding disorders, Hx of haemorrhagic CVA, intracranial disease (neoplasm/aneurysm/AVM), severe HTN, ↓Pt, ↑INR **B**.
Caution: ↑risk of bleeding (e.g. drugs, recent bleeding/trauma/procedures)[BNF], **L** (avoid if severe), **H** (if severe), **R/P**.
SE: bleeding, nausea, fever, ↓Pt (reversible).
Monitor: FBC.
Dose: 400 *nanograms*/kg/min for 30 min, then 100 *nanograms*/kg/min for ≥48 h (continue for 12–24 h post-PCI), for max of 108 h. Needs concurrent heparin (LMWH is simplest, and patients are usually already on this).

Specialist use only: get senior advice or contact on-call cardiology.

TOLBUTAMIDE

Oral antidiabetic (short-acting sulphonylurea).
Use/CI/Caution/SE: as glibenclamide, but shorter action and hepatic metabolism* means ↓risk of hypoglycaemia,

esp in elderly/RF* (↓reliance on renal excretion). Can also ⇒ headache.

Interactions: corticosteroids and rifampicin ↓ its fx. NSAIDs, chloramphenicol, sulphonamides, fluconazole and miconazole ↑ its fx. β-blockers mask 'hypos'. (Mild **W+**).

Dose: 0.5–2.0 g daily in divided doses, with food.

TOLTERODINE/DETRUSITOL

Antimuscarinic, antispasmodic.

Use: detrusor instability (urinary incontinence, frequency or urgency).

CI/Caution/SE: as oxybutynin (mostly antimuscarinic fx; see p. 174), **P/B**.

Dose: 1–2 mg bd po. (MR preparation available as 4 mg od po; not suitable if RF or LF).

tPA (= tissue-type Plasminogen Activator) see Alteplase.

TRAMADOL

Opioid analgesic: also ↓s pain by ↑ing 5HT/adrenergic transmission.

Use: moderate pain (esp musculoskeletal).

CI/Caution/SE: as morphine, but ↓respiratory depression, ↓constipation, ↓addiction. Rarely ⇒ Ψ disturbances.

Dose: 50–100 mg up to 4-hourly po (or im/iv). Postoperatively; initially 100 mg im/iv, then 50 mg every 10–20 min to max total dose of 250 mg in 1st h, then prn (max 600 mg/day).

TRANEXAMIC ACID

Antifibrinolytic: ↓s fibrinolysis.

Use: bleeding: acute bleeds[1] (esp 2° to anticoagulants, thrombolytic/anti-Pt agents, epistaxis, haemophilia), menorrhagia[2], hereditary angioedema[3].

CI: TE disease, **R** (if severe).

Caution: gross haematuria (can clot and obstruct ureters), DIC, **P**.

SE: GI upset, colour vision Δs, TE.

Dose: 15–25 mg/kg bd/tds po (if severe, 0.5–1 g tds iv)[1]; 2–4.5 g/day po in 2–4 divided doses[2,3].

TRIAMTERENE

K^+-sparing diuretic (weak).

Action/Use/CI/Caution/SE: as amiloride, but $\Rightarrow$ less $\downarrow$BP $\therefore$ not used for HTN (unless used with other drugs).

Warn: urine may go blue.

Interactions: $\uparrow$s lithium levels. NSAIDs $\uparrow$risk of RF and $\uparrow K^+$.

Dose: almost exclusively used with stronger K^+-wasting diuretics in combination preparations (e.g. co-triamterzide). For doses on its own, see BNF.

☠ Beware if on other drugs that $\uparrow K^+$, e.g. amiloride, spirono-lactone, ACE-i, angiotensin II antagonists and ciclosporin. Do not give with oral K^+ tablets or dietary salt substitutes. ☠

TRI-IODOTHYRONINE

See Liothyronine; synthetic T_3.

TRIMETHOPRIM

Antifolate antibiotic ('static'): inhibits dihydrofolate reductase.

Use: UTIs (rarely other infections).

CI: blood disorders (esp megaloblastic $\downarrow$Hb).

Caution: $\downarrow$folate (or predisposition to), porphyria, R/P/B/E.

SE: see co-trimoxazole (Septrin), but much less frequent and severe (esp BM suppression, skin reactions). Also **GI upset**, rash, rarely other hypersensitivity.

Interactions: $\uparrow$s (nephro)toxicity of ciclosporin and $\uparrow$s phenytoin levels. (Mild **W+**).

Dose: 200 mg bd po (100 mg nocte for chronic infections or as Px if at risk; NB: risk of $\downarrow$folate if long-term Rx).

TROPICAMIDE EYE DROPS

Antimuscarinic: mydriatic (short-acting, weak), cycloplegic.

Use: eye examination.

Caution: $\uparrow$IOP.

SE: blurred vision, $\downarrow$accommodation. Rarely precipitation of glaucoma ($\uparrow$risk if > 60 yrs and long sighted).

Dose: 1 drop of 0.5 or 1.0% solution.

VALPROATE

Antiepileptic and mood stabiliser: potentiates and ↑s levels of inhibitory neuropeptide GABA.

Use: epilepsy (also mania but as valproate *semisodium*[BNF]).

CI: porphyria, personal or family Hx of severe liver dysfunction, **L**.

Caution: SLE, ↑bleeding risk*, R, P (⇒neural-tube/craniofacial dfx), B.

SE: **sedation**, **cerebellar fx** (see p. 175; esp tremor, ataxia), **headache, GI upset**, ↑Wt, SOA, alopecia, skin reactions, ↓cognitive/motor function, Ψ disorders, encephalopathy (2° to ↑NH_4). Rarely but seriously **hepatotoxicity, blood disorders** (esp ↓Pt*), **pancreatitis** (mostly in 1st 6 months of Rx).

Warn: of clinical features of pancreatitis and liver/blood disorders.

Monitor: LFTs.

Interactions: fx ↓d by antimalarials (esp mefloquine), anti-depressants, antipsychotics and some antiepileptics[BNF]. Mild **W+**.

Dose: initially 300 mg bd, ↑ing to max of 2.5 g/day.

Can give false-positive urine dipstick for ketones.

VALSARTAN/DIOVAN

Angiotensin II antagonist.

Use: HTN.

CI: biliary obstruction, cirrhosis, **L** (if severe)/**P/B**.

Caution/SE/Interactions: see Losartan.

Dose: initially 40–80 mg od, ↑ing if necessary to maintenance of 80–160 mg od.

VANCOMYCIN

Glycopeptide antibiotic. Poor po absorption (unless bowel inflammation*), but still effective against C. *difficile*** as acts 'topically' in GI tract.

Use: serious Gram-positive infections[1] (inc endocarditis Px and systemic MRSA), AAC[2] (give po)

Caution: Hx of deafness, IBD* (only if given po), R/P/B/E.

otoxicity, ototoxicity (stop if tinnitus develops), **isorders, rash, hypersensitivity** (inc anaphylaxis, skin reactions), nausea, fever, phlebitis/irritation at ction site. Also shock or rash/flushing of upper body if given oo rapidly iv.

Monitor: serum levels: keep predose trough levels 5–10 mg/l; start monitoring after 3rd dose (1st dose if RF). Also U&Es, FBC, urinalysis (and auditory function if elderly/RF).

Dose: 1 g bd ivi over 100 min[1] (↓dose in elderly); 125 mg qds po[2].

VENLAFAXINE/EFEXOR

Serotonin and **N**oradrenaline **R**euptake **I**nhibitor (SNRI): antidepressant with ↓ sedative/antimuscarinic fx cf TCAs.

Use: depression, anxiety disorder.

CI: L/R (if either severe), **P/B**.

Caution: Hx of mania, seizures, glaucoma or cardiac disease.

SE: GI upset, ↑**BP** (dose-related; monitor BP if dose >200 mg/day), **withdrawal fx** (common even if doses only a few hours late), **rash** (consider stopping drug, as can be 1st sign of severe reaction*), insomnia/agitation, dry mouth, sexual dysfunction, drowsiness, dizziness, headache.

Warn: report rashes*.

Interactions: ☠ *Never give with MAOIs.* ☠ (Mild **W+**.)

Dose: 37.5–150 mg bd po; start low and ↑ dose if required. Efexor XL MR od preparation available (max 225 mg od).

VENTOLIN see Salbutamol; β2 agonist bronchodilator.

VERAPAMIL

Ca^{++} channel blocker (rate-limiting type): fx on heart (⇒ ↓HR, ↓contractility*) >vasculature (dilates peripheral/coronary arteries); i.e. reverse of the dihydropyridine type (e.g. nifedipine). Only Ca^{++} channel blocker w useful antiarrhythmic properties (class IV).

Use: HTN[1], angina[2], arrhythmias (SVTs, esp instead of adenosine if asthma[3]).

CI: ↓BP, ↓HR (<50 bpm), 2nd-/3rd-degree HB, SAN block, SSS, AF/flutter 2° to WPW, porphyria **H*** (inc Hx of).

Caution: AMI, 1st degree HB, **L/P/B**.

SE: constipation (rarely other GI upset), HF, ↓**BP** (dose-dependent), HB, headache, dizziness, fatigue, ankle oedema, hypersensitivity, skin reactions.

Interactions: ↑risk of AV block and ↓HR with ☠ **β-blockers** ☠ and amiodarone. ↑s hypotensive fx of anaesthetics and antihypertensives. ↑s fx of digoxin, theophyllines, carbamazepine and ciclosporin. Rifampicin ↓s its fx.

Warn: fx ↑d by grapefruit juice (avoid).

Dose: 80–160 mg tds po[1]; 80–120 mg tds po[2]; 40–120 mg tds po[3]; 5–10 mg iv (over ≥2 min w ECG monitoring), followed by additional 5 mg iv if necessary after 5–10 min[3].

VIAGRA see Sildenafil; phosphodiesterase inhibitor.

VOLTAROL see Diclofenac; moderate-strength NSAID.

WARFARIN

Oral anticoagulant: blocks synthesis of vitamin-K-dependent factors (II, VII, IX, X) and proteins C and S.

Use: Rx/Px of TE; see pp. 154–8.

CI: severe HTN, PU, bacterial endocarditis, **P**.

Caution: recent surgery, **L/R/B**.

SE: haemorrhage, rash, fever, diarrhoea. Rarely other GI upset, 'purple-toe syndrome', skin necrosis, hepatotoxicity, hypersensitivity.

Warn: fx are ↑d by alcohol.

Dose: see pp. 155–7.

☠ NB: **W+** and **W−** denote significant interactions throughout this book: take particular care with antibiotics and drugs that affect cytochrome **P450** (see p. 176). ☠

XALATAN see Latanoprost; topical PG analogue for glaucoma.

ZANTAC see Ranitidine; H$_2$ antagonist.

FIRLUKAST/ACCOLATE

ukotriene receptor antagonist.
Use: asthma (non-acute).
CI: L/B.
Caution: Churg–Strauss syndrome, **R/P/E**.
SE/Monitor: as Montelukast, but ↑**hepatotoxicity**, **W+**.
Dose: 20 mg bd po.

ZESTRIL see Lisinopril; ACE-i.

ZIDOVUDINE (AZT)

Antiviral (nucleoside analogue): reverse-transcriptase inhibitor.
Use: HIV Rx (and Px, esp of vertical transmission).
CI: severe ↓NØ or ↓Hb (caution if other blood disorders), **B**.
Caution: ↓B_{12}, ↑ risk of lactic acidosis, **L/R/P/E**.
SE: blood disorders (esp ↓Hb or ↓WCC), **GI upset, headache, fever**, taste Δs, sleep disorders. Rarely hepatic/pancreatic dysfunction, myopathy, seizures, other neurological/Ψ disorders.
Interactions: paracetamol ↑s risk of blood disorders.
Dose: see BNF.

ZIRTEK see Cetirizine; non-sedating antihistamine for allergies.

ZOPICLONE

Short-acting hypnotic (cyclopyrrolone): potentiates GABA pathways via same receptors as benzodiazepines (although isn't a benzodiazepine!): can also ⇒ dependence* and tolerance.
Use: insomnia (not long-term*).
CI: respiratory failure, sleep apnoea, MG, **L** (if severe**), **P/B**.
Caution: Ψ disorders, Hx of drug abuse*, **R/E**.
SE: *all rare:* GI upset, taste Δs, behavioural/Ψ disturbances (inc psychosis, aggression), hypersensitivity.
Dose: 7.5 mg nocte, ↑ing to 12.5 mg if necessary. If LF (non-severe**), RF or elderly give 3.75 mg. .

ZOTON see Lansoprazole; PPI.

ZYBAN see Buproprion; adjunct to smoking cessation.

L/R/H = Liver, Renal and Heart failure (full key see p. x)

Drug selection

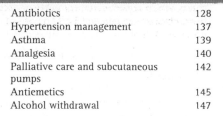

Antibiotics	128
Hypertension management	137
Asthma	139
Analgesia	140
Palliative care and subcutaneous	142
pumps	
Antiemetics	145
Alcohol withdrawal	147

ANTIBIOTICS

IMPORTANT POINTS

- The following *are only guides to a rational start to Rx.*
  Local organisms, sensitivities and prescribing preferences vary
  widely: if unsure, consult your microbiology department/
  pharmacy.
- Empirical (best-guess) Rx is given unless stated otherwise.
- When deciding whether 'severe' treatment is necessary, consider
  each individual's comorbidity and whether you have time to
  give simple Rx first and then add on or change if patient is not
  improving.
- Get as many appropriate cultures as possible *before* starting Rx.

> ☠️It is essential to ask each patient *in person* about allergies
> before prescribing any antibiotics. Do not rely on notes or drug
> charts, which are often not complete or accurate. Remember:
> *if you prescribe it, you are liable!* If patient is unconscious, check
> notes thoroughly (or contact relatives/GP if time). Do not let an
> incident (or near-incident) be the way you learn this! ☠️

PNEUMONIA

1. Community-acquired pneumonia

> *Adverse prognostic features of community-acquired pneumonia*
> Adapted with permission of BMJ group from BTS guidelines.
> *Thorax* 2001; **56** (suppl IV).
> *Core features (CURB):*
>
> **C**onfusion (MTS <8/10)
> **U**rea >7 mmol/l
> **R**espiratory rate >30/min
> **B**P: systolic <90 mmHg, ±diastolic <60 mmHg
>
> *Pre-existing features:*
> Age >50 years
> Coexisting disease(s)

Additional features:
> Hypoxia: PaO_2 <8 kPa (or sats <92%) on any FiO_2
> Bilateral or multilobe involvement

- *≥2 core:* admit as severe/life-threatening: consider HDU/ITU.
- *1 core or 0 core and pre-existing features:* decide on admission using clinical judgement with aid of other prognostic features.
- *no adverse features:* admission not necessary on clinical grounds (but social circumstances and patient's wishes should be considered).

Treatment:

Mild: amoxicillin 500 mg tds po ± erythromycin 500 mg qds po.
Severe: co-amoxiclav 1.2 g tds iv + erythromycin 500 mg qds iv.
+ flucloxacillin 1 g qds iv if *S. aureus* (Hx or epidemic of 'flu).
+ rifampicin 600 mg bd po/iv if *Legionella* (do urinary Ag test).

- If no improvement, change co-amoxiclav to 2nd-generation cephalosporin (e.g. cefuroxime 0.75–1.5 g tds iv).
- If risk factors, consider Rx for aspiration or TB as below.
- If penicillin hypersensitivity, use erythromycin only.

Causes of community-acquired pneumonia (UK adults)
Adapted with permission of BMJ group from Lim, W.S. *et al.*
Thorax 2001; **56**: 296–301.

- 48% *Streptococcus pneumoniae:* esp in winter or living in shelters/prison.
- 23% **viruses:** influenza (A ≫ B), RSV, rhinoviruses, adenoviruses.
- 15% *Chlamydia psittaci:* esp from animals, but only 20% from birds (less commonly *Chlamydia pneumoniae*, esp if long-term Hx and headache).
- 7% *Haemophilus influenzae.*

> 3% ***Mycoplasma pneumoniae:*** ↑s during 4-yearly epidemics.
> 3% ***Legionella pneumophila:*** ↑d if recent travel (esp Turkey, Spain).
> 2% ***Moraxella catarrhalis:*** ↑d in elderly.
> 1.5% ***Staphylococcus aureus:*** mostly post-influenza ∴ ↑s in winter.
> 1.4% **Gram-negative infection:** *E. coli, Pseudomonas, Klebsiella, Proteus, Serratia.*
> 1.1% **Anaerobes:** e.g. bacteroides, fusobacterium, *Gemella.*
> 0.7% ***Coxiella burnetii:*** ↑s in April–June and in sheep farmers.
>
> NB: 25% are mixed aetiology (accounts for total of >100%).
> In ⩾20%, causative pathogen is not identified.

The term 'atypical pathogens' is not considered useful by the
BTS (refers to *Mycoplasma, Chlamydia, Coxiella, Legionella*).
There is no characteristic clinical presentation for the pneumonias
they cause.

2. Hospital-acquired pneumonia
Mild: co-amoxiclav 625 mg tds po.
Severe: 3rd-generation cephalosporin, e.g. ceftriaxone 1 g od iv
(max 4 g/day) or cefotaxime 1 g bd iv (max 2 g qds). Ceftazidime
1 g tds iv (max 2 g tds) can be used if complicated infection
(see below), if *Pseudomonas* suspected or if failure to improve.
± metronidazole 500 mg tds iv if aspiration suspected.
± gentamicin if septic shock or failure to improve.
MRSA: teicoplanin/vancomycin if confirmed colonisation
/infection.

> *Causes of hospital-acquired pneumonia*
> Reproduced with permission from Hammersmith Hospitals NHS
> Trust Clinical Management Guidelines & Formulary 2001.
>
> * ***Simple:*** (w/in 7 days of admission): *H. influenzae, S. pneumoniae,
>   S. aureus,* Gram-negative organisms (see top of page).
> * ***Complicated*:*** Gram-negative organisms (esp *P. aeruginosa*),
>   *Acinebacter,* MRSA.
> * ***Anaerobic**:*** *Bacteroides, Fusobacterium, Gemella.*

- *Special situations:*
  1 Head trauma, coma, DM, RF: consider *S. aureus*.
  2 Mini-epidemics in hospitals: consider *Legionella*.

*>7 days after admission, recent multiple antibiotics or complex medical Hx (e.g. recent
ITU/recurrent admissions or severe comorbidity).

**esp if risk of aspiration, recent abdominal surgery, bronchial obstruction/poor dentition.

3. Aspiration pneumonia

Treatment as for community- or hospital-acquired pneumonia,
+ metronidazole 500 mg tds po/iv.

4. Cavitating pneumonia

Co-amoxiclav 1.2 g tds iv + flucloxacillin 1 g qds iv.
 NB: need to exclude TB with sputum/Heaf test ± pleural Bx.

> 'TANKS' cause cavitation: TB, *Aspergillus*, *Nocardia*, *Klebsiella*,
> *S. aureus* (and *pSeudomonas*).

TB

Get expert advice from respiratory/microbiology departments.
NB: contact consultant in communicable disease control.
 Rx normally comes in two phases:

- *Initial phase:* for 1st 2 months: ↓s bacterial load and covers all
  strains: ethambutol** + Rifater* (rifampicin + isoniazid +
  pyrazinamide).
- *Continuation phase:* for next 4 months: Rifanah* or Rimactazid*
  (rifampicin + isoniazid). If resistance to rifampicin/isoniazid
  known (or suspected), continue pyrazinamide.

- Combined tablets* ⇒ ↑compliance and ease of prescribing.
- All doses are by weight; see BNF for details.
- All are hepatotoxic: check LFTs before and during Rx.
- **Ethambutol** is nephrotoxic and can ⇒ optic neuritis:** check
  U&Es and visual acuity before and during Rx. Alternative is

streptomycin (also nephrotoxic), but both can be omitted if ↓risk of isoniazid resistance.

ACUTE BRONCHITIS

Rx not usually needed in previously healthy patients <60 years old.

- *COPD:* 1st-line: amoxicillin 500 mg tds po/iv.
             2nd-line: co-amoxiclav, erythromycin or doxycycline.
- *Bronchiectasis:* cefuroxime 750 mg tds iv (co-amoxiclav po if mild).
- *Cystic fibrosis:* ciprofloxacin 500 mg bd po (or 400 mg bd ivi)
  if *Pseudomonas* suspected. Otherwise try gentamicin + piperacillin
  until sensitivities known.

UPPER RESPIRATORY TRACT AND ENT INFECTIONS

- *Acute epiglottitis:* cefotaxime 1 g tds iv ± metronidazole 500 mg
  tds iv (ceftriaxone alone should suffice in children).
- *'Strep throat':* penicillin V 500 mg qds po; consider only if local
  pus, severe systemic features, ↓immunity or no improvement
  after 3 days.
- *Sinusitis/otitis media:* amoxicillin 500 mg tds po if local pus or if
  does not resolve in 2–3 days (as would expect if viral aetiology).
- *Otitis externa:* mostly bacterial; give topical Sofradex or
  Otomize. Less commonly fungal (look for black spores); give
  topical Otosporin or Neo-cortef. If does not resolve or
  evidence of perichondritis (inflamed pinna), cellulitis, boils
  or local abscess, refer to ENT for specialist advice and
  consideration of systemic Rx (e.g. amoxicillin, co-amoxiclav,
  flucloxacillin) and local toilet (esp if fungal).

URINARY TRACT INFECTIONS

- *Simple UTI:* trimethoprim 200 mg bd po. Another option is
  nitrofurantoin 50 mg qds po (not suitable if RF).
- *Pyelonephritis (suspect if loin pain/systemic features):* cefotaxime
  1 g tds iv. If no response within 24 h (and still no culture results),
  try ampicillin 1 g qds iv + gentamicin.

> **Causes of UTIs**
>
> Mnemonic = 'SEEK Pee Pee':
>
> *S. aureus** (*S. saprophyticus, S. epidermis* ↑d in women).
>
> *E. coli:* 70–80% of cases (penicillin resistance common).
>
> *Enterococci**, e.g. *Streptococcus faecalis.*
>
> *Klebsiella***
>
> *Proteus mirabilis***
>
> *Pseudomonas.*
>
> Others: *Candida* (esp if urinary catheter), *Serratia.*
>
> *↑d if renal stones or recent instrumentation (e.q. cystoscopy)
>
> **↑d if renal stones, recent instrumentation, obstructive uropathy or recurrent infections.

GI INFECTIONS

Gastroenteritis

- Simple infections rarely need Rx; contact microbiology department if in doubt.
- *AAC (Clostridium difficile):* metronidazole 400 mg tds po and *stop other antibiotics if possible*. If no response after 6 days, change to vancomycin 125 mg qds po for 7–10 days.

H. pylori eradication: 'triple therapy'

1 wk of Rx sufficient is in 90% of cases (some give 2-wk courses).

1   *Antibiotic 1.* amoxicillin 1g bd po.
2   + *Antibiotic 2:* clarithromycin 500 mg bd po (or metronidazole 400 mg tds if previous eradication failure).
3   + *Acid suppressant:* PPI (e.g. lansoprazole 30 mg bd) or ranitidine bismuth citrate 400 mg bd (NB: ≠ 'normal' ranitidine!).

Lansoprazole is available in combination packs with amoxicillin + clarithromycin as *Heliclear*, and with clarithromycin + metronidazole as *Helimet*: simpler to prescribe and ↑compliance.

MALARIA

Clues: fevers (±3-day cycles ± rigors), ↓Pt, ↓Hb, jaundice, ↑spleen/liver, travel (even >1 year previously).

Always consult infectious diseases ± microbiology team if malaria suspected/confirmed.

If confirmed non-falciparum ('benign'):

- Chloroquine: initial dose 600 mg po, then 300 mg 6–8 h later, then 300 mg od 24 h later for 2 days (all doses of chloroquine as *base*). Consider following with primaquine if *P. ovale* or *P. vivax*.

If falciparum ('malignant') or species mixed/unknown:
If seriously ill (e.g. ↓GCS), get senior help and give:

- Quinine: load* with 20 mg/kg ivi (maximum 1.4 g) over 4 h. After 8–12 h, give 10 mg/kg (maximum 700 mg) iv over 4 h bd/tds for up to 7 days (↓doses to 5–7 mg/kg if RF or >48 h iv Rx needed), changing to 600 mg tds po once able to swallow and retain tablets to complete a 7-day course.
- Fansidar: if quinine resistance known or suspected, give 3 tablets as single dose following the course of quinine (each tablet = pyrimethamine 25 mg + sulfadoxine 200 mg). Doxycycline 200 mg od po for ≥7 days is used instead if Fansidar resistance.
- Consider artesunate or artemether: get specialist advice.

If stable, normal GCS, and able to swallow and retain tablets:

- Quinine: 600 mg tds po for 7 days (followed by Fansidar or doxycycline as above).

☠Quinine doses here are as **salt** (specify this on prescription): do not confuse with **base**, which has different doses. *Do not give iv loading dose if quinine, quinidine or mefloquine given in past 24h.

MENINGITIS

Empirical Rx (until results of LP known – esp Gram stain).

- Cefotaxime 2 g qds ivi: Rx of choice for *N. meningitides* (aka meningococcus), by far the most common cause in UK adults.

Consider:

- Ampicillin 2 g 4 hourly iv + gentamicin iv if *Listeria* suspected, e.g. immunosuppression or indicative CSF: non-TB Gram-positive bacilli.
- Aciclovir 10 mg/kg over 1 h tds iv if HSV encephalitis suspected, e.g. more prominent confusion, behavioural Δs and seizures.
- TB Rx as for pneumonia: if risk factors or suggestive CSF findings (↑LØ, ↑protein, ↓glucose).

Causes of meningitis in the UK

Common:
- *N. meningitidis*, serotype B: majority (70–80%) of cases.
- *N. meningitidis*, serotype C: ↓ing secondary to vaccine.
- *N. meningitidis*, serotype A: ↑ing again (had been ↓ing).
- *S. pneumoniae*: stable incidence.

Rarer:
- Gram-negative bacilli.
- *Listeria monocytogenes*: esp neonates, age >60, ↓immunity.
- *H. influenzae*, type b: ↓ing secondary to vaccine.

Don't forget:
- Viral: HSV/HZV, EBV, HIV, mumps: esp if encephalitic (↓GCS). Less commonly entero/echo/coxsackie/polio viruses.
- TB, other bacteria, e.g. *Borrelia*: esp if ↓immunity/HIV.
- Fungi: cryptococcus, candida: esp if ↓immunity/HIV.
- Group B *Streptococcus*: predominantly in neonates.
- *S. aureus*: if neurosurgery, ↓immunity, invasive lines, IVDU.

EYE INFECTIONS

For conjunctivitis, blepharitis* and corneal abrasions:

- chloramphenicol 1 drop (or ointment application to lids*) qds. ± doxycycline po if systemic Rx required*. Consult opthalmologist for advice if at all unsure (extra care needed if contact lens wearer).

CELLULITIS

Mild (e.g. Venflon site infection): co-amoxiclav 375 mg tds po.
Severe: benzylpenicillin 1.2 g 4–6 hourly + flucloxacillin 1 g qds iv.
+ metronidazole 500 mg tds iv if suspect anaerobes, e.g. abdominal wound.
+ consider vancomycin if confirmed MRSA colonisation/infection.

BONE AND JOINT INFECTIONS

Osteomyelitis: suspect in any postoperative joint or deep DM ulcer.

- Flucloxacillin 1 g qds iv + fusidic acid 500 mg* tds iv
  (*6–7 mg/kg if weight <50 kg).

Septic arthritis: suspect if sudden-onset pain/inflammation.

- Treatment as osteomyelitis, but consider changing after
  urgent Gram stain, e.g. to iv 3rd-generation cephalosporin
  (e.g. cefotaxime, ceftriaxone) if *H. influenzae* suspected
  (Gram-negative bacilli, esp in children). Suspect *Salmonella*
  in sickle cell disease or TB/fungi if immunocompromised.

PUO

No routine antibiotics indicated, but suspect and exclude abdominal abscess, TB, Ca (esp abdominal/haematological) and other causes.

> ### Causes of PUO
> - Faulty thermometer!
> - Abdominal abscess: liver, subphrenic, pelvic.
> - Other infection: UTI, TB, malaria, SBE, virus (EBV, CMV, HIV).
> - Autoimmune: rheumatoid arthritis, Still's disease, PMR, sarcoid, PAN, SLE/connective tissue disease.
> - Cancer: lymphoma, leukaemia, solid tumours (esp abdominal).
> - Drugs: almost any (inc drugs of abuse), often assoc w ↑EØ.
> - Other: PEs, haematomas, alcoholic hepatitis, FMF.
> NB: up to 25% of cases remain unexplained.

NEUTROPOENIA

If temperature >37.5°C for >2 h and no clues as to the fever's aetiology, give:

- *For 1st/2nd episodes:* gentamicin 5 mg/kg od iv + Tazocin 4.5 g tds iv (use ceftazidime 2 g tds iv if penicillin allergy).
- *For subsequent episodes (if treated as above):* meropenem 1 g tds iv + vancomycin 1 g bd iv (and get expert help).

> NB: always do full septic screen before Rx: blood, urine and any other appropriate cultures (e.g. sputum, stool, central/other lines) ± CXR.

HYPERTENSION MANAGEMENT

Adapted with permission from Brown, M.J. British Hypertension Society guidelines. *Journal of Human Hypertension* 2003; **17**: 81–6.

Treat if: systolic >160 mmHg and/or diastolic >100 mmHg (or >140/90 mmHg if other cardiovascular risk or target organ damage, i.e. hypertensive retinopathy (haemorrhages, exudates, papilloedema), MI, ischaemia, dissecting aneurysm, pulmonary oedema, encephalopathy, seizures, coma, ARF).
Aim for: systolic <140 mmHg and diastolic <85 mmHg (<80 mmHg if DM; this probably also applies to other high cardiovascular risk groups, e.g. post-stroke, renal disease).
Primary causes: look for and exclude (esp if treatable), e.g. RAS, Cushing's, Conn's (primary hyperaldosteronism), phaeo (esp if variable BP, headaches, sweats, palpitations).
NB: stress (inc 'white-coat HTN') and drug withdrawal (esp alcohol) are common temporary causes.

Important points:

- Make lifestyle modifications first: ↓salt, ↓Wt, ↓alcohol, stop smoking, ↑exercise, ↑fruit/vegetables.
- Make a *written* Rx plan for (other) doctors, nurses and patient. Include target BP and how Rx should change if it is not achieved.

- Age/ethnic origin influence response to drugs (see table below).
- A single agent is rarely successful at achieving target BP. Rather than ↑ing doses, add 2nd and 3rd agents, which often work in an additive or complementary fashion, esp if table below used.

CHOICE OF DRUG: RATIONAL COMBINATION THERAPY ('CAMBRIDGE AB/CD RULE')

Step	Younger (<55 years) and non-black	Older (>55 years) or black*
1	A or B	C or D
2	A (or B**) + C or D	C or D + A (or B**)
3	A + C + D	C + D + A
4	Resistant hypertension***	Resistant hypertension***

*African (not Asian) origin. **B is less preferred here, as could mean combination of two diabetogenic drugs (e.g. β-blocker + diuretic), esp in elderly. ***Add α-blocker, spironolactone or other diuretic ± specialist referral and consider missed primary cause or poor compliance.

☺ good for. ⊘ avoid/caution. ☠ beware!

A = ACE-i, e.g. enalapril initially 5 mg od (2.5 mg if elderly or RF). ☺ HF, DM, CRF (*with caution!*). ⊘ PVD. ☠ Pregnancy, bilateral RAS (∴ must check U&Es 2 wks after starting, esp if vasculopathy or existing renal impairment).
  Angiotensin II receptor blockers can also be used but are normally reserved for when ACE-i not tolerated (esp dt dry cough).
B = β-blocker, e.g. atenolol 25 mg bd. ☺ anxious, IHD. ⊘ HF, dyslipidaemia, PVD, if on verapamil/diltiazem. ☠ asthma/COPD, HB.
C = Ca⁺⁺ channel blocker: dihydropyridines such as amlodipine 5 mg or nifedipine LA (e.g. Adalat LA 20–30 mg od) usually 1st-line ⊘ oedema ☠ aortic stenosis, recent ACS. If IHD 'rate limiting' types (verapamil, diltiazem) often preferred. ☠ HF, HB, if on other rate limiting drugs (esp β-blockers).
D = diuretic, e.g. bendroflumethiazide 2.5 mg od. ☺ oedema. ⊘ dyslipidaemia. ☠ gout.

NB: only starting doses are given; see main drugs section or BNF for doses thereafter.

When to change Rx (after checking compliance first!):

- BP <5 mmHg lower: switch category of drug (i.e. from A or B to C or D).
- BP >5 mmHg lower but:
  - drug not tolerated: swap within category (i.e. from A to B, or from C to D).
  - still suboptimal: either ↑dose or add 2nd agent (often better).

ASTHMA

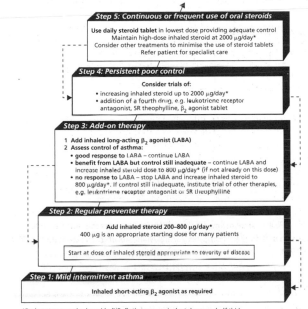

Step 5: Continuous or frequent use of oral steroids

Use daily steroid tablet in lowest dose providing adequate control
Maintain high-dose inhaled steroid at 2000 µg/day*
Consider other treatments to minimise the use of steroid tablets
Refer patient for specialist care

Step 4: Persistent poor control

Consider trials of:
- increasing inhaled steroid up to 2000 µg/day*
- addition of a fourth drug, e.g. leukotriene receptor antagonist, SR theophylline, β_2 agonist tablet

Step 3: Add-on therapy

1 Add inhaled long-acting β_2 agonist (LABA)
2 Assess control of asthma:
- **good response to LABA** – continue LABA
- **benefit from LABA but control still inadequate** – continue LABA and increase inhaled steroid dose to 800 µg/day* (if not already on this dose)
- **no response to LABA** – stop LABA and increase inhaled steroid to 800 µg/day*. If control still inadequate, institute trial of other therapies, e.g. leukotriene receptor antagonist or SR theophylline

Step 2: Regular preventer therapy

Add inhaled steroid 200–800 µg/day*
400 µg is an appropriate starting dose for many patients

Start at dose of inhaled steroid appropriate to severity of disease

Step 1: Mild intermittent asthma

Inhaled short-acting β_2 agonist as required

*Beclometasone or budesonide (NB: fluticasone equivalent doses are half this).

Figure 1 BTS guidelines for management of asthma in adults. Adapted with permission of BMJ group from *Thorax* 2003; **58** (suppl 1): 24.

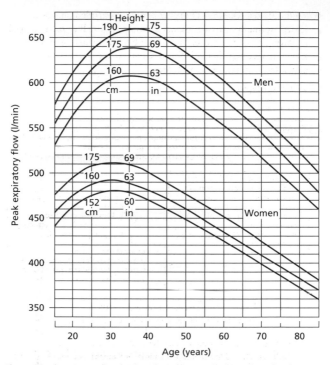

Figure 2 Peak expiratory flow (PEF) predictor for normal adults. Adapted with permission of BMJ group from Gregg, I. and Nunn, A.J. *British Medical Journal* 1989; **298**: 1098.

ANALGESIA

Important points for postoperative patients:

- Oral route often ineffective *for all operations* (due to gastric stasis).

- Epidural anaesthesia (EDA) and patient-controlled analgesia (PCA) normally provide maximal opiates (as well as other drugs) ∴ beware of giving more. Try strong NSAID as below and get advice from anaesthetist if this does not work.
- Consider local/regional anaesthesia.

Choice of analgesic:

General rules
- Look for/treat reversible causes and reassess cause at each step.
- Regular Rx ↓s relapses *but always review to check whether still needed.*
- If pain ↓s, step down and ensure adequate pm analgesia in case ↑s again.
- Pain is rarely refractory to the correct Rx and has many adverse medical fx.
- If pain persists, get senior or specialist help (e.g. anaesthetist or pain team).

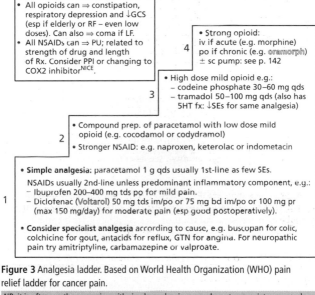

- All opioids can ⇒ constipation, respiratory depression and ↓GCS (esp if elderly or RF – even low doses). Can also ⇒ coma if LF.
- All NSAIDs can ⇒ PU; related to strength of drug and length of Rx. Consider PPI or changing to COX2 inhibitor^{NICE}.

4
- Strong opioid:
  iv if acute (e.g. morphine)
  po if chronic (e.g. oramorph)
  ± sc pump: see p. 142

3
- High dose mild opioid e.g.:
  – codeine phosphate 30–60 mg qds
  – tramadol 50–100 mg qds (also has 5HT fx: ↓SEs for same analgesia)

2
- Compound prep. of paracetamol with low dose mild opioid (e.g. cocodamol or codydramol)
- Stronger NSAID: e.g. naproxen, ketorolac or indometacin

1
- **Simple analgesia:** paracetamol 1 g qds usually 1st-line as few SEs.

  NSAIDs usually 2nd-line unless predominant inflammatory component, e.g.:
  – Ibuprofen 200–400 mg tds po for mild pain.
  – Diclofenac (Voltarol) 50 mg tds im/po or 75 mg bd im/po or 100 mg pr (max 150 mg/day) for moderate pain (esp good postoperatively).

- **Consider specialist analgesia** according to cause, e.g. buscopan for colic, colchicine for gout, antacids for reflux, GTN for angina. For neuropathic pain try amitriptyline, carbamazepine or valproate.

Figure 3 Analgesia ladder. Based on World Health Organization (WHO) pain relief ladder for cancer pain.

NB: it is often worth persevering with simple analgesia even when strong opiates are used as they have additive fx in combination (esp in combination with paracetamol).

PALLIATIVE CARE AND SUBCUTANEOUS PUMPS

- Underprescribed dt stigma of being a 'final measure': ensure good communication with patient, relatives and nurses as to reasons for use.
- Gives smooth symptom control, esp for pain, but also useful for other symptoms, e.g. nausea, xs secretions, agitation. Good if unable to take po medications, avoids cannulation, only single 24-h prescription needed (no delays in drug administration on busy wards).
- Palliative care, Macmillan and hospital pain teams will help if unsure of the indications or how to set up these pumps.

CONTENTS

1 *Diamorphine:* calculate dose needed for 24-h prescription from the past 24 hours' requirements (if variable, look at longer-term trend). If taking other opioids, use the following *rough* guide:

$$1\,mg\ diamorphine\ sc\ = 3\ \text{mg morphine po}$$
$$= 15\ \text{mg tramadol po}$$
$$= 25\ \text{mg pethidine im}$$
$$= 35\ \text{mg codeine po/im}$$

(For conversion from fentanyl, see its entry in main drugs section.)

NB: this table applies only for the specific route(s) of each drug stated, as bioavailability can vary widely with routes. Also, it does not take into account duration of action, although this can be ignored if 24-h requirements for each drug are calculated.

2 Antiemetic: choose from (*generally start at lowest dose*):
- Metoclopramide 30–100 mg/24 h: normally 1st choice (esp for promotility fx to counter opioid constipation; but CI if GI obstruction!).
- Haloperidol 2.5–5 mg/24h: good general antiemetic.

- Levomepromazine 6.25–12.5 mg/24 h. Good if cause unknown or multifactorial. Use ↑doses (25–50 mg/24 h) if sedation required.

3 *Optional extras:*
- Drugs to ↓respiratory secretions:
  - glycopyrronium 0.6–1.2 mg/24 h: becoming more popular.
  - hyoscine hydrobromide 0.6–2.4 mg/24h: normally sedative but can ⇒ paradoxical agitation.
- Sedatives, e.g. midazolam 20–100 mg/24h if restlessness or agitation is the solitary symptom or refractory to levomepromazine. Care/↓dose if elderly, respiratory depression, benzodiazepine-naive.

Compatibility of drugs in syringe drivers
It is advised that only two or three drugs are used per syringe driver. All antiemetics listed above are compatible with diamorphine. For addition of 'optional extras', see table below; for all other combinations, check with the hospital pharmacy or drug information office. Out-of-hours authoritative information on compatibility (and other palliative care prescribing issues) can be found at the excellent website www.palliativedrugs.com.

Compatibility* of specific three-drug combinations: diamorphine and antiemetic and one other 'optional extra' drug.

Diamorphine *plus*	Glycopyrronium	Hyoscine *hydrobromide*	Midazolam
Metoclopramide	Not recommended	Not recommended	Compatible*
Haloperidol	Not known	Compatible*	Compatible*
Levomepromazine	Compatible*	Compatible*	Compatible*

*Compatibility is restricted to usual dose ranges of the drugs.

EXAMPLE PRESCRIPTION

Prescribe each drug individually in the 'regular prescriptions' section of the drug chart, as shown here:

DATE/ TIME	INFUSION FLUID	VOL-UME	ADDITIVES IF ANY DRUG AND DOSE	RATE OF ADMIN	DURA-TION	DR'S SIGNATURE	TIME START-ED	TIME COMP-LETED	SET UP BY SIG-NATURE	BATCH No.
08/01	Water for injection	48 ml	+ Diamorphine 60 mg	TN						
			+ Metoclopramide 30 mg							
	Total of 48 ml to run subcutaneously via syringe driver at 2 ml per hour over 24 h									

Figure 4 Example drug chart of diamorphine subcutaneous pump. *NB: 60 mg diamorphine/24 h is **example dose**; individual patient needs vary (see p. 142).*

GENERAL POINTERS IN CHRONIC PAIN/ PALLIATIVE CARE

- *Laxatives:* give with opiates as Px rather than later as Rx.
- *Fentanyl patches:* smooth pain control w/o multiple injections or tablets (just change patch every 3rd day). Also less constipating.
- *Breakthrough analgesia:* always write up in case regular medications become insufficient. Oral opiates (e.g. Oramorph) often best; 1/6th of regular 24-h opiate equivalent dose is usually sufficient.
- *Simple analgesia:* do not forget as often effective, e.g. paracetamol.
- *Steroids:* consider for nausea, as pain adjuvant (esp liver capsule pain), and for short-term Rx of ↓appetite: get specialist help.
- *Always consider new causes of pain/distress*, esp if patient unable to give Hx: often treatable, iatrogenic or can be disguised/made worse by more analgesia, e.g. opiate-induced constipation, patient positioning, UTI, urinary retention, mental anguish (esp 'unfinished business'), pathological fractures.

!!

> *Commonly missed problems*
> - ↑Ca^{++}: esp consider if confusion and constipation (other symptoms: 'bones, stones, groans and psychic moans'); see p. 191 for Mx.
> - *Spinal cord compression:* ↑back pain, sensory/sphincter disturbance, limb weakness – *can be treated* with immediate high-dose steroids (e.g. dexamethasone phosphate 12–16 mg iv then 8 mg po bd) and radiotherapy.

ANTIEMETICS

General rules

- Look for/treat reversible causes (see below).
- Reassess causes at each step.
- Start iv/im (and switch to po ASAP).
- Consider sc pump if chronic (see p. 142).
- Don't stop Rx unless cause removed.

> Designed for cancer patients where refractory nausea common. Steps 3 and 4 rarely necessary in other settings.

4
- ↑Levomepromazine.
- Consider octreotide or dexamethasone.

3
- Try levomepromazine or a 5HT₃ antagonist (e.g. ondansetron).

2
- Try alternative or add 2nd narrow-spectrum agent.
- Consider dexamethasone if cause is brain tumour (or other cause of ↑ICP) or chemotherapy.

1
- Start narrow-spectrum (1st line) drug: choose most appropriate agent from the table on next page.

Figure 5 Antiemetic ladder.

Causes of nausea

- *Drugs:* esp opiates, chemotherapy. Commonly also dopamine agonists, NSAIDs, digoxin.
- *GI:* constipation, but also surgical (obstruction, peritonism) and medical (oesophagitis, gastritis, PU) causes.
- *Neurological:* migraine, ↑ICP (esp meningitis, tumour).
- *Metabolism:* ↑Ca⁺⁺ (also ↓Na⁺, ↑K⁺), organ failure.
- *Infection:* gastroenteritis but also UTI, respiratory infections.
- *Other:* pregnancy, MI (esp inferior, often ↓pain if DM or elderly).

Commonly used 1st line/narrow-spectrum antiemetics (see also Palliative care section, pp. 142–4).

Class	Example	Good for	Beware
Phenothiazine (D_2 antagonist)	**Prochlorperazine** 10–20 mg po or 12.5 mg im (Stemetil)	Opiates, general anaesthetic, postoperative, chemo/radiotherapy (if mild)	⇒ ↑prolactin, extrapyramidal fx, ↓s seizure threshold, ↓BP
Benzamine (D_2 antagonist)	**Metoclopramide** 10 mg tds po/im/iv (Maxolon)	GI causes (↑s GI motility*), migraine, drugs (esp opiates)	⇒ ↑prolactin, extrapyramidal fx, CI if GI obstruction*
Benzamine (D_2 antagonist)	**Domperidone** 10–20 mg tds po or 30–60 mg tds pr (not iv or im)	Parkinson's disease**, morning-after pill, chemotherapy	⇒ ↑prolactin, but minimal sedation and extrapyramidal fx**
Antihistamines	**Cyclizine** 50 mg tds po/im/iv	GI obstruction*/postoperative N&V, vestibular/labyrinthine disorders	⇒ Antimuscarinic fx (esp sedation). Avoid in IHD (↓s beneficial cardiodynamic fx of opiates)
5HT₃ antagonists	**Ondansetron** 8 mg bd po/im/iv (16 mg od pr) **Granisetron** **Tropisetron**	Severe/resistant cases (esp chemotherapy)	Minimal side effects: headache, constipation, dizziness

ALCOHOL WITHDRAWAL

A 'detox' programme comprises the following components:

SEDATION

↓s anxiety and risk of DTs(= delirium tremens)/seizures. Benzo-diazepines are often used, esp in tapered regimes, e.g. as follows:

Alcohol withdrawal regime. With permission from Prof. H. Ghodse, Liaison Psychiatry Department, St. George's Hospital.

Day	Diazepam	Chlordiazepoxide
1	15 mg qds	30 mg qds
2	10 mg qds	30 mg tds
3	10 mg tds	20 mg tds
4	5 mg qds	20 mg bd
5	5 mg tds	10 mg bd
6	5 mg bd	10 mg od
7	5 mg od	10 mg prn

> **The above are only suggested initial average regimes.** *Dose requirements vary considerably* with patient size and previous experience (tolerance) of benzodiazepines. Regular review of these doses and writing up prn doses is strongly recommended. Only start once acute intoxication has resolved.

VITAMINS

> ***Wernicke's encephalopathy***
> Triad of ophthalmoplegia, ataxia and confusion (also ⇒ ↓BP, ↓temperature, nystagmus, ↓GCS). NB: often missed!

If Wernicke's known, suspected or anticipated (e.g. severe chronic abuse), give high-dose vitamins B and C at Rx doses:

- Pabrinex 1 & 2 (= pair of vials) bd iv*/im for 2 days, then 1 pair daily for 5 days, continue until clinical improvement stops.

For all patients give:

- Pabrinex 1 & 2: 1 pair od iv*/im for 3–5 days as Px (unless receiving Rx as above).
- Thiamine (vitamin B_1): 100 mg tds po for $\geq$2 wks.
- Multivitamins: 1 tablet/day, long-term.

!! ☠If giving Pabrinex iv*, must give over at least 10 min. If giving iv or im, have resuscitation facilities at hand (can $\Rightarrow$ anaphylaxis). ☠

MAINTENANCE OF ABSTINENCE

Must:

- Encourage abstinence and refer to local addiction services.
- Treat depression and try to arrange adequate social support.

Consider the following as aids:

- *Acamprosate:* ↓s pleasurable fx of alcohol.
- *Disulfiram:* causes unpleasant symptoms if patient drinks alcohol.
- *Naltrexone:* ↓s craving and relapse rate.

How to prescribe

Insulin	150
Anticoagulants	154
Thrombolysis	161
Controlled drugs	163

INSULIN

TYPES

Many exist, with differences in the timing of action onset (O), peak (P) and duration (D).

For acute use, e.g. DKA and sliding scales, inc perioperative:

- Soluble (aka normal/neutral) can be given **iv** (and **sc** as other types), e.g. Actrapid, Humulin S:

  iv: O/P immediate, D 0.5 h;   **sc:** O 0.5–1 h, P 2–4 h, D 8 h.

For maintenance use, i.e. normal chronic control (sc only):

- **Aspart (▼ NovoRapid), lispro** (Humalog): recombinant human analogues. Rapid onset ⇒ ↑eating flexibility (can give immediately before meals; other types of sc must be given 30 min before), ↓duration ⇒ fewer hypos (esp before meals). O 0.25 h, P 1–3 h, D 2–5 h.
- **Isophane**: mixed with protamine to ↑action duration, e.g. Insulatard, Humulin I (=i). O 0.5–2 h, P 2–12 h, D 18–24 h. Often given with varying proportions of soluble (shorter-acting) forms to make 'biphasic' preparations, which ⇒ smoother 24-h control, e.g. Mixtard, Humulin M3. 30% soluble and 70% isophane is the most common mixture used (the soluble percentage is always the one specified in the name, e.g. Mixtard 30, Humulin M3).
- **Insulin zinc suspension** (IZS): slowest onset and longest action. 'Mixed' (e.g. Humulin Lente, Monotard) or 'crystalline' forms (e.g. Humulin Zn, Ultratard). O 2–4 h, P 6–24 h, D 20–28 h.
- **▼Glargine**: new, long-acting recombinant insulin with delayed and prolonged absorption from sc injection site ⇒ constant, more 'physiological' basal supply; can give od in evening (e.g. Lantus).

SLIDING SCALES

For optimal blood glucose control in diabetics if (i) DKA/HONK, (ii) preoperative/NBM, (iii) MI*/ACS*, (iv) severe concurrent illness (e.g. sepsis).

For MI*/ACS*, ivi of glucose + insulin + K⁺ often preferred (aka GIK, DIGAMI). Use local protocols if they exist; can often be found in CCU/A&E.

Example of how to write an insulin sliding scale on a drug chart

DATE/ TIME	INFUSION FLUID	VOL- UME	ADDITIVES IF ANY DRUG AND DOSE	RATE OF ADMIN	DURA TION	DR'S SIGNATURE	TIME START- ED	TIME COM- PLETED	SET UP BY SIG NATURE	BATCH No.
08/01	Normal saline	50 ml	Actrapid 50 units	No bolus		TN				
08/01	Glucose saline	1 litre								
		CBG (= BM)	INSULIN ivi (ml/h)							
		0–4	0.5 (+ call Dr if CBG <2.5)							
		4.1–7	1							
		7.1–9	2							
		9.1–11	3							
		11.1–13	4							
		≥13.1	6							
Always run glucose saline ivi at 125 ml per hour if CBG (BM) <15.										

Figure 6 Drug chart, showing slide scale.

These are average requirements and ∴ only a suggested *initial* regime: requirements will vary widely between individuals and within an individual over time (esp with intercurrent illness, e.g. infections). Regular review and adjustment is essential – see pp. 152–3 for how to do this.

Important points
- Check Venflon is working before adjusting sliding scale (may be reason why BG not falling).
- prn insulin (e.g. 2–5 units actrapid sc) can be used when estimated requirements not sufficient. NB: ☠ risk of

hypoglycaemia. ☠ Use only when review not possible and if experienced nurses available. Risk can be ↓d by writing on chart that duty doctor must be called to instruct on exact dose to be given. Beware of patients with unpredictable responses to insulin and if patient not known to you.

- Always give glucose* saline (4% glucose and 0.18% saline) ivi at 125 ml/h when CBG <15. If RF or mild HF give 5% glucose* ivi at a slower rate. If severe HF give 10% glucose* (preferably via central line) at 60–70 ml/h. KCl should be added according to individual needs (see pp. 167–8). Write up 50% glucose iv prn in case of severe hypoglycaemia.

- State clearly to nursing staff the frequency with which CBGs are required: very sick patients (e.g. DKA/HONK) need CBGs every half-hour and ideally regular laboratory glucose readings (more accurate). If not very sick and CBGs stable (e.g. preoperative), 2–4-hourly usually suffices.

- Stop oral hypoglycaemics and adjust for residual effects they may be having. Remember to reintroduce before stopping sliding scale!

*NB: glucose = dextrose. Low-strength glucose solutions used to be called dextrose solutions; this is now being phased out.

Amount of insulin: initial doses and adjustment

Prescribe 50 units of soluble insulin (Actrapid or Humulin S) in 50 ml normal saline to run via a syringe driver according to one of the regimes (A, B, C, D) below:

1 Start with regime A, unless severe insulin resistance (i.e. normally takes ≥100 units sc insulin/day), in which case start with B.
2 If BG >10 (or >7 during acute MI, where target BG even lower) for 3 consecutive hourly tests and is ↑ing (or ↓ing by <25% in the past hour), step up to next sliding scale (i.e. if on A, step up to B; if on B, step up to C, etc.).
3 If BG <3.5 mmol/l, step down to next scale (i.e. if on B, step down to A; if on C, step down to B, etc.).

Table showing suggested insulin ivi regimes

CBG (= BM)	Insulin ivi (units/h)			
	Regime A	Regime B	Regime C**	Regime D**
0.0–4.0*	0.5	0.5	0.5	0.5
4.1–7.0	1	2	3	4
7.1–9.0	2	4	6	8
9.1–11.0	3	6	9	12
11.1–13.0	4	8	12	16
>13.0	6	12	18	24

*Stop ivi for 15 min if severe hypoglycaemia (CBG <2.5 or symptoms) and give Rx as on p. 188.
Otherwise treat more gently with 5–10% glucose ivi and maintain insulin infusion (esp if DKA).
**Rarely needed; used mostly for patients with severe insulin resistance (i.e. on more than 100
units insulin/day before admission).
Reproduced with permission from Prof. S. Kumar, Dr. A. Rahim and Dr. P. Dyer, Endocrinology
Department, University of Warwick Medical School.

Coming off a sliding scale

Consider once eating/drinking normally and CBGs normal/stable:

- If post-DKA, change back only if urine free of ketones (ideally,
  blood ketones should also be checked) and pH back to normal.
- If postoperative and no reason to suppose change in needs
  (i.e. no infection), go straight back to preoperative regime.
- Avoid hypos by continuing ivi until 1st sc dose starts to work
  (usually 10–30 min). Always change from iv to sc before a meal.

The following is only a guide to how to start sc regimes (always
consult your hospital's diabetes team if unsure):

1 Calculate daily requirements by doubling the number of units
  used in the past 12 h from the sliding scale.
2 Start qds sc regime. If patient is well and CBGs very stable, this
  step may be omitted (i.e. go straight to a bd regime). Give 1/3rd
  of total daily dose at 10pm (as intermediate insulin e.g. Humulin I (i)
  or Insulatard), then give the rest (as short-acting insulin e.g.
  Actrapid or Humulin S) divided equally between
  pre-breakfast, pre-lunch and pre-evening meal doses.
3 Start bd sc regime: give 60% of daily dose pre-breakfast and
  the remaining 40% pre-evening meal, both doses as biphasic
  30/70 insulin (e.g. Humulin M3 or Mixtard 30).

PREOPERATIVE GUIDELINES: GENERAL POINTS (FOR ALL PATIENTS)

Local protocols should be used if they exist, otherwise a sensible way to progress would be to:

- Ensure patient 1st on operating list and fast from midnight*.
- Stop all long-acting insulins the night before the operation.
- Withhold all DM medications for morning of operation.
- Prescribe 5 or 10% glucose ivi in case of hypoglycaemia.
- Proceed as per table below:

*If pm-only list, give light breakfast and normal morning medications (but no intermediate/long acting insulins), monitor CBG 1–2-hourly. Start sliding scale/GIK at 11am (unless well controlled type II) or if CBGs uncontrolled.

Type of surgery	Type II (control good)	Type I and type II (control poor/fasting glucose >10)
	Monitor CBGs 2-hourly	Monitor CBGs 1-hourly
Minor: expect to eat normally the same day	After operation give normal medications ASAP with a meal (sliding scale not usually required).	Start sliding scale/GIK at 10pm the night before op. Give normal medications and meal ASAP after op.
Major/GI: not expected to eat the same day	Start sliding scale/GIK if CBGs not controlled**. Convert back to normal medications once CBGs stable and eating/drinking normally.	Start sliding scale/GIK at 10pm the night before op. Convert back to normal medications once CBGs stable and eating/drinking normally.

**Uncontrolled CBGs = single reading >15 or consistently >10.

ANTICOAGULANTS

WARFARIN

Consult your hospital anticoagulant service if ever unsure about indications, doses or interactions. Refer as early before discharge as practicable so outpatient monitoring is arranged in time.

Basics

Oral anticoagulant for long-term Rx/Px of TE: loading usually takes several days, so heparin (quicker-acting) is short-term cover until therapeutic levels are achieved.

Monitoring

Via INR = patient's PT (prothrombin time) compared to that of a control. A target INR is set at the start of Rx, according to indication (see below); variations of ± 0.5 are acceptable.

BSH guidelines for target INRs. Adapted with permission from *British Journal of Haematology* 1998; **101**: 374–87.

Indication	Target INR
DVT/PE[1]	2.5
Thrombophilia (if symptomatic)[2]	2.5
AF (or other causes of cardiac emboli[3])	2.5
Bioprosthetic heart valves[4]	2.5
Mechanical heart valves	3.5

[1] If recurrent DVT/PE *whilst on therapeutic Rx*, target INR = 3.5.
[2] Antiphospholipid syndrome is an exception with target INR = 3.5.
[3] Dilated cardiomyopathy, mural thrombus post-MI, rheumatic valve disease and/or for 6 wks before elective DC cardioversion.
[4] Only for first 3–6 months post-insertion at discretion of each centre.

Although not yet in the BSH guidelines, a target INR of 2.5 is widely agreed for nephrotic syndrome (generally once albumin <25 g/l).

> Always put target INR clearly next to the prescription on drug chart: on call doctor will not know target (esp if not 2.5). Patient's 'yellow book' (anticoagulation record) documents an individual's target INR if you are unsure.

Starting Rx

Check INR before 1st dose and every day for 1st week, then assess stability of INR and scale down sensibly. If on heparin, do not stop until 2 days after therapeutic INR achieved.

For loading regimes, where possible use your hospital's own guidelines, since these often vary. Otherwise, it is sensible to use the BSH guidelines:

arfarin loading regime. Adapted with permission of BMJ group from Fennerty, A. et al. *British Medical Journal* 1984; **288**: 1268–70.

Day 1		Day 2		Day 3		Day 4	
INR	Dose (mg)	INR	Dose (mg)	INR	Dose (mg)	INR	Dose* (mg)
<1.4	10	<1.8	10	<2.0	10	<1.4	>8
		1.8	1	2.0–2.1	5	1.4	8
		>1.8	0.5	2.2–2.3	4.5	1.5	7.5
				2.4–2.5	4	1.6–1.7	7
				2.6–2.7	3.5	1.8	6.5
				2.8–2.9	3	1.9	6
				3.0–3.1	2.5	2.0–2.1	5.5
				3.2–3.3	2	2.2–2.3	5
				3.4	1.5	2.4–2.6	4.5
				3.5	1	2.7–3.0	4
				3.6–4.0	0.5	3.1–3.5	3.5
				>4.0	0	3.6–4.0	3
						4.1–4.5	Miss 1 day then 2 mg
						>4.5	Miss 2 days then 1 mg

*Predicted maintenance dose.

!! ■■

Situations when doses (especially loading) may need review
↓**doses if:** age >80 years, LF, HF, post-op, ↑baseline INR or taking drugs that potentiate warfarin (check for **W+** symbols in this book).
↑**doses if:** taking drugs that inhibit warfarin (check for **W−** symbols in this book).
Herbal remedies: can have significant interactions – always ask patients directly if taking any, as they may not realise the importance. Check each one with your hospital's drug information office for significance.
Alcohol and diet: can affect dosing, especially if intake varies – the goalposts will move for an individual's therapeutic range.
It is a common misconception that BMI influences response.

NB: there is evidence that loading with 5 mg for the 1st 3 days achieves therapeutic levels as quickly with less overshoot, and practice may soon change to reflect this. The latest British Society for Haematology guidelines (due for review in 2004) can be viewed at www.bcshguidelines.com.

If interrupting warfarin (e.g. before operation/procedure), do not reload post-op as above, but restart at double usual dose for 2 days, then return to usual dose *if no contraindications* (e.g. bleeding/taking **W+** drugs).

> Make small infrequent dose changes unless INR dangerously high or low. 'Steering a supertanker' is a good analogy, as there is often significant delay between dose changes and their fx.

Overtreatment/poisoning

> *Seek expert help from haematology on-call* as xs vitamin K can make re-anticoagulation difficult, as fx can last for weeks ∴ ⇒ ↑risk from condition that warfarin was started for.

Recommendations for management of excess warfarin (BSH guidelines). Adapted with permission from *British Journal of Haematology* 1998; **101**: 374–87.

INR	Action
3.0–6.0 if target 2.5 (4.0–6.0 if target 3.5)	• ↓dose or stop warfarin, restart when INR <5.0
6.0–8.0 and no/minor bleeding	• Stop warfarin; restart when INR <5.0
>8.0 and no/minor bleeding	• Stop warfarin; restart when INR <5.0 • Vitamin K 0.5–2.5 mg po if other bleeding risks, e.g. age >70 years, Hx of bleeding complications or liver disease
Major bleeding, e.g. ↓ing Hb or cardiodynamic instability	• Stop warfarin • Vitamin K 5 mg po/iv (repeat 24 h later if necessary) • FFP 15ml/kg or prothrombin complex concentrate 50 units/kg

Warfarin and surgery

Warfarin is often stopped 4–5 days ahead of surgery and other invasive procedures ($\pm$ heparin cover until day of procedure). Exact protocol depends on procedure involved and risks of coming off warfarin: get senior advice from team doing the procedure $\pm$ haematologists if at all unsure.

Warfarin and pregnancy

Warfarin is contraindicated in early pregnancy (teratogenic during weeks 6–12). Women of childbearing age must be warned of the potential risks and to seek expert haematology advice if planning a pregnancy.

HEPARIN

For immediate and short-term Rx/Px of TE. Two major types: low-molecular-weight heparins and unfractionated heparin.

Low-molecular-weight heparins (LMWHs)

Given sc. ↑Convenience (↓monitoring, can give to outpatients). ↓Incidence of HIT* and osteoporosis cf unfractionated heparin means now preferred for most indications (esp MI/ACS, DVT/PE, Rx and pre-cardioversion of AF). Dalteparin (Fragmin), enoxaparin (Clexane) and tinzaparin (Innohep) are the most commonly used; each hospital tends to use one in particular; ask nurses which one they stock or call pharmacy.

Monitoring
Via anti-Xa assay: usually necessary only if renal impairment (i.e. creatinine >150), pregnancy or at extremes of Wt (i.e. <45 kg or >100 kg). Take sample 3–4 h post dose.

!! HIT* = heparin-induced thrombocytopoenia. It is not uncommon and can occur with all heparins. Watch for ↓ing platelet count. Get senior help if concerned. If confirmed, stop heparin immediately.

Unfractionated heparin

Given iv*: quickly reversible (immediately if protamine given; see p. 161), which makes it useful in settings where desired amount of anticoagulation may change rapidly, e.g. perioperatively, if patient at ↑risk of bleeding, or if using extracorporeal circuits such as cardiopulmonary bypass and haemodialysis. Also used with recombinant fibrinolytics in AMI.

Can be given sc (only for Px), but now largely replaced by LMWH.

Monitoring

Via APTT ratio (= **A**ctivated **P**artial **T**hromboplastin **T**ime of patient divided by that of control serum). APTT is less commonly called KCCT. Results can (rarely) be given as patient's exact APTT: the normal range is 35–45 s. You then need to calculate the ratio: take the middle of the normal range of (i.e. 40 s) for your calculations. *Target ratio is commonly 1.5–2.5,* but this can vary: check your hospital's protocol and aim for the middle of range. NB: there is no national (let alone international) consensus on methods of measuring APTT, so results are not yet standardised.

Starting iv treatment

1 *Load with 5000** units as iv bolus*: prescribed on the 'once-only' section of the drug chart (give 10 000** units if severe PE).
2 Set up ivi at 15–25 units/kg/h: usually = 1000–2000 units/h. A sensible starting rate is 1500 units/h, which can be achieved by adding 25 000 units of heparin to 48 ml of normal saline to make 50 ml of solution (500 units/ml), which runs at 3 ml/h via a syringe driver. This can be written up as follows:

DATE/ TIME	INFUSION FLUID	VOLUME	ADDITIVES IF ANY DRUG AND DOSE	RATE OF ADMIN	DURA- TION	DR'S SIGNATURE	TIME START- ED	TIME COM- PLETED	SET UP BY SIG- NATURE	BATCH No.
08/01	Normal saline	50 ml	Heparin 25,000 units			TN				
	run at 3 ml per hour as ivi									

Figure 7 Drug chart, showing how to write up heparin infusion.

NB: dosing for co-therapy with fibrinolytics (according to ESC guidelines) is slightly different; see p. 163.

Check APTT ratio after every 6 h, then every 6–10 h until stable, and then daily at a minimum, adjusting to the following regime:

APTT ratio	Action
<1.2	Give 5000-unit bolus iv and ↑ivi by 200–250 units/h
1.2–1.5	Give 2500-unit bolus iv and ↑ivi by 100–150 units/h
1.5–2.5	No change
2.5–3.0	↓ivi by 100–150 units/h
>3.0	Stop ivi for 1 h then restart ivi, ↓ing by 200–250 units/h

This regime is based on APTT *ratio* therapeutic range of 1.5–2.5. *Don't take sample from drip arm* (unless from site distal to ivi).

Adjustments are safest made by writing a fresh ivi prescription at a different strength, but the same effect can also be achieved by calculating the appropriate rate change to the original prescription.

Variable rate of ivi (for fixed prescription of 25 000 units heparin in 50 ml saline)

Desired heparin ivi rate (units/h)	Rate of ivi (ml/h)	Desired heparin ivi rate (units/h)	Rate of ivi (ml/h)
1000	2.0	1500	3.0
1050	2.1	1550	3.1
1100	2.2	1600	3.2
1150	2.3	1650	3.3
1200	2.4	1700	3.4
1250	2.5	1750	3.5
1300	2.6	1800	3.6
1350	2.7	1850	3.7
1400	2.8	1900	3.8
1450	2.9	1950	3.9

Overtreatment/poisoning (all heparins)

If significant bleeding, stop heparin and observe: iv heparin has short $t_{1/2}$ (30 min–2 h), so fx wear off quickly. If bleeding continues or is life-threatening, consider iv protamine (1 mg per 80–100 units of heparin to be neutralised as ivi over 10 min. ↓doses if giving >15 min after heparin stopped). NB: protamine is less effective against LMWH, and repeat administration may be required.

Seek expert help from haematology on-call if in any doubt!

THROMBOLYSIS

INDICATIONS

From Resuscitation Council (UK) guidelines 2000.

- Onset of chest pain <12 h + Hx compatible with MI + one of:
  - ST elevation >2 small squares in 2 adjacent chest leads
  - ST elevation >1 small square in ≥2 limb leads
  - new LBBB: must assume it is new if cannot prove is old
  - posterior infarct (ST depression + dominant R wave in V1–3)
- Onset of chest pain 12–24 h ago and evidence of an evolving infarct, e.g. ongoing chest pain or worsening ECG changes.

☠CONTRAINDICATIONS☠

From ESC guidelines 2003 (with permission from *European Heart Journal* 2003; **24**: 28–66). Local guidelines/checklists often exist and should be used if available: consult cardiology ± haematology on-call if in any doubt.

Absolute

- Haemorrhagic stroke or stroke of unknown origin at any time.
- Ischaemic stroke in past 6 months.
- CNS damage or neoplasms.
- Major trauma, head surgery/injury (w/in 3 weeks).
- GI bleeding (w/in past month).
- Known bleeding disorder.
- Aortic dissection.

Relative

- TIA in past 6 months.
- Oral anticoagulant therapy.
- Pregnancy or w/in 1 week postpartum.
- Non-compressible punctures.
- Traumatic resuscitation.
- Refractory HTN (systolic >180 mmHg).
- Advanced liver disease.
- Infective endocarditis.
- Active PU.

CHOICE OF AGENT

Always use your hospital's protocol if one exists – contact CCU, A&E or look on your hospital intranet for details.

Choose between streptokinase and a recombinant thrombolytic such as alteplase, reteplase or tenecteplase (each hospital tends to stock one in particular).

NICE guidance (due for review Oct 2005) recommends that, in hospitals, the choice of agent should take account of:

- *'The likely balance of benefit and harm (e.g. stroke) to which each of the thrombolytic agents would expose the individual patient.'* Recombinant forms (cf. streptokinase) are probably more efficacious and have ↓incidence of allergic reactions, CCF and bleeding other than stroke. However they have ↑ incidence of haemorrhagic stroke.
- *'Current UK clinical practice, in which it is accepted that patients who have previously received streptokinase should not be treated with it again.'* Streptokinase is less effective and more likely to cause allergic reaction after first administration (due to Ab production). Don't give if patient has been given it in the past.
- *'The hospital's arrangements for reducing delays in the administration of thrombolysis.'* Some agents are quicker to set up and administer and this can reduce 'door to needle times'.

> ### Heparin co-therapy
> Recombinant forms always need concurrent iv heparin for
> 24–48 h (*this does not normally apply for streptokinase*). Use your
> hospital's A&E/CCU protocol if one exists. Otherwise use *ESC
> guidelines:* 60 units/kg (max 4000 units) iv bolus, then ivi at
> 12 units/kg/h for 24–48 h (max 1000 units/h). Monitor APTT at 3, 6,
> 12, 24 and 48 h, with target APTT ($\neq$ APTT *ratio!*) of 50–70 s. NB:
> this is different to 'standard' iv heparin regimes (see pp. 159–60).

Side effects

Commonly bleeding (mostly mild and at iv sites; if severe or suspect
CVA, stop ivi and get senior help), N&V, ↓BP (improves if
transiently ↓ rate of ivi and raise legs), mild hypersensitivity (inc
uveitis). Rarely anaphylaxis, GBS.

CONTROLLED DRUGS

In reality, this only concerns prescriptions for strong opiates,
although not necessary for codeine, DF118, dextropropoxyphene
or tramadol.

The following must be written in the *doctor's own handwriting*:

- Date: may be stamped but *not* computer-generated.
- Full name and address of patient.
- Drug name plus its form* (and, where appropriate, strength).
- Dosing regimen.
- Total amount of drug to be dispensed *in words and figures*.

*Omitting the form is a common reason for an invalid prescription.
It is often assumed to be obvious from the prescription (e.g. fentanyl
as a patch or Oramorph as a liquid), but it still has to be written.

Benzodiazepines (and barbiturates, although used very rarely now)
are also controlled, but the above prescribing requirements do not
apply.

Miscellaneous

Intravenous fluids	166
Steroids	169
Sedation/sleeping tablets	171
Benzodiazepines	173
Side-effect profiles	174
Cytochrome P450	176

INTRAVENOUS FLUIDS

CRYSTALLOIDS

Isotonic: used mostly for maintenance (replacement) regimes:

- *Normal (0.9%) saline:* 1 l contains 150 mmol Na^+.
- *5% glucose*:* 1 l contains 278 mmol (=50 g) glucose, which is immediately metabolised and included only to make the fluid isotonic (calories are minimal, at 220 kcal). Used as method of giving pure H_2O and as ivi with insulin sliding scales to avoid hypoglycaemia (see pp. 150–4).
- *Glucose* saline:* 1 l contains mixture of NaCl (30 mmol Na^+) and glucose (4% = 222 mmol). Useful as contains correct proportions of constituents (excluding KCl, which can be added to each bag) for average daily requirements (see below). Suboptimal long term, as does not account for individual patient needs (esp if these are far from average).

Non-isotonic: used less commonly; mostly specialist situations only:

- *Hypertonic (5%) saline:* 1 l contains 750 mmol Na^+; given mostly for severe hyponatraemia. ☠ Seek specialist help first. ☠
- *Hypotonic (0.45%) saline:* for severe ↑Na^+ (e.g. HONK).
- *10% and 20% glucose*:* for mild/moderate hypoglycaemia.
- *50% glucose:* for severe hypoglycaemia (see p. 188) and if insulin being used to lower K^+ (see p. 190).

*NB: glucose = dextrose. Low-strength glucose solutions used to be called dextrose solutions; this is now being phased out.

COLLOIDS (= plasma substitutes/expanders)

- Gelofusine or Haemaccel: both are gelatin-based and used in resuscitation of shock (non-cardiogenic). NB: the electrolyte contents are often overlooked: 1 l Gelofusine has 154 mmol Na^+; 1 l Haemaccel has 145 mmol Na^+ + 5.1 mmol K^+.
- *Hartmann's solution:* compound sodium lactate, used in surgery/trauma (also 1 l contains 5 mmol K^+).

STANDARD DAILY REQUIREMENTS

$= 3\,l\,H_2O$, 40–70 mmol K^+, 100–150 mmol Na^+.

If no oral intake (preoperative, $\downarrow$GCS, unsafe swallow, post-CVA, etc.), this can be provided as follows:

DATE/ TIME	INFUSION FLUID	VOL- UME	ADDITIVES IF ANY DRUG AND DOSE	RATE OF ADMIN	DURA- TION	DR'S SIGNATURE	TIME START- ED	TIME COM- PLETED	SET UP BY SIG- NATURE	BATCH No.
08/01	5% Glucose	1 l	20 mmol KCl		8°	TN				
08/01	Normal saline	1 l			8°	TN				
08/01	5% Glucose	1 l	20 mmol KCl		8°	TN				

Figure 8 Drug chart, showing how to write up intravenous fluids.

This '2 sweet (5% glucose), 1 sour (0.9% saline)' regime is commonly used in fit preoperative patients. If in any doubt, normal (0.9%) saline is generally safest, unless liver failure (see below) or if Na^+ outside normal range ($\downarrow$ or $\uparrow$). Always get senior help if unsure: incorrect fluids can be as dangerous as any other drug.

Individual requirements may differ substantially according to:

- Body habitus, age, residual oral intake, if on multiple iv drugs (which are sometimes given with significant amounts of fluid).
- Insensible losses (normally about 1 l). $\uparrow$skin losses in fever/burns. $\uparrow$lung losses in hyperventilation/inhalation burns.
- GI losses (normally about 0.2 l). Any vomiting ($\uparrow Cl^-$ content) or diarrhoea ($\uparrow K^+$ content) must be taken into account as well as less obvious causes, e.g. ileus, fistulae.
- Fluid compartment shifts, esp vasodilation in sepsis and anaphylaxis.

These points seem obvious but are easy to forget!

K^+ CONSIDERATIONS

Do not give >10 mmol/h unless K^+ dangerously low, when it can be given quicker (see p. 191). Surgical patients often need less K^+ in

1st 24 h post-op, as K^+ is released by cell death ($\therefore$ proportional to extent of surgery).

IMPORTANT POINTS

- *Take extreme care if major organ failure:*
  - *Heart failure:* heart can quickly become 'overloaded' and $\Rightarrow$ acute LVF. Even if not currently in HF, beware if predisposed (e.g. Hx of HF or IHD).
  - *Renal failure:* unless pre-renal cause (e.g. hypovolaemia), do not give more fluid than residual renal function can deal with. Seek help from renal team if at all concerned; good fluid Mx greatly influences outcomes in this group.
  - *Liver failure: **should not receive any saline**;* always use 5% glucose. Serum Na^+ may be $\downarrow$d, but total body Na^+ is often $\uparrow$d. Any saline will work its way into the wrong compartment (e.g. peritoneal fluid $\therefore$ $\uparrow$ing ascites).
- If in doubt, give fluid challenges: small volumes (normally 200–500 ml) of fluid over short periods of time, to see whether clinical response to BP, urine output or left verticular function is beneficial or detrimental before committing to longer-term fluid strategy.
- In general, encourage oral fluids: homeostasis (if normal) is safer, less expensive and less consuming of doctor/nurse time than iv fluids. Beware if $\downarrow$swallow, fluid overload (esp if HF or RF), pre-/post-operative or if homeostasis disorders (esp SIADH).
- Check the following before prescribing any iv fluids:
  - *Clinical markers of hydration:* skin turgor/temperature, mucous membranes, JVP, peripheral oedema, pulmonary oedema. Often overlooked and very useful!
  - *Recent input and output:* if at all concerned, ask nurses for strict fluid balance chart. Daily weights are often very informative, esp if doubts over accuracy of fluid charts.
  - Recent U&Es, esp K^+.

It can be difficult to illicit all this information under time pressure. The trick is to know when to take extreme care. Be particularly careful if you do not know the patient when on call, and be wary when asked to 'just write up another bag' without reviewing the patient. Often, you will be asked to prescribe fluids when no longer necessary or even when they may be harmful. To save time for those on call (and to ↑ the chances of your patients getting appropriate fluids), leave clear instructions with the nurses and on the drug chart for as long as can be sensibly predicted (esp over weekends/long holidays).

STEROIDS

CORTICOSTEROIDS

Equivalent dose	Main uses
Prednisolone 5 mg	Acute asthma/COPD, rheumatoid arthritis (po)
Methylprednisolone 4 mg	Acute flares rheumatoid arthritis/MS (iv)
Dexamethasone 750 μg	↑ICP, CAH, Dx Cushing's (iv/po)
Hydrocortisone 20 mg	Acute asthma/COPD (iv)

Mineralocorticoid fx for these are all mild (apart from hydrocortisone) and minimal with dexamethasone (hence its use where H_2O and Na^+ retention are particularly undesirable).

Side effects = Cushing's syndrome!
- *Metabolic:* Na^+/fluid retention*, hyperlipoproteinaemia, leukocytosis, negative K^+/Ca^{++}/nitrogen balance, generalised fluid/electrolyte abnormalities.
- *Endocrine:* hyperglycaemia/↓GTT (can ⇒ DM), adrenal suppression.
  - *Fat*:* truncal obesity, moon face, interscapular ('buffalo hump') and suprascapular fat pads.
  - *Skin:* hirsutism, bruising/purpura, acne, striae, ↓healing, telangiectasia, thinning.

– *Other:* impotence, menstrual irregularities/amenorrhoea,
↓growth (children), ↑appetite*.
- *GI:* pancreatitis, peptic/oesophageal ulcers: give PPI if on
↑doses.
- *Cardiac:* HTN, CCF, myocardial rupture post-MI, TE.
- *Musculoskeletal:* proximal myopathy, osteoporosis, fractures (can
⇒ avascular necrosis).
- *Neurological:* ↑epilepsy, ↑ICP/papilloedema (esp children on
withdrawal of corticosteroids).
- *Ψ:* mood Δs (↑ or ↓), psychosis (esp at ↑doses), dependence.
- *Ocular:* cataracts, glaucoma, corneal/scleral thinning.
- *Infections:* ↑susceptibility, ↑speed (↑severity at presentation),
TB reactivation, ↑risk of chickenpox/shingles/measles.

> SEs are dose-dependent. If patient is on high doses, make sure this
> is intentional: it is not rare in fluctuating (e.g. inflammatory)
> illnesses for patient to be left on high doses by mistake. Seek
> specialist advice if unsure.

Cautions
Can mostly be worked out from the SEs. Caution should be taken if
patient already has a condition that is a potential SE.
NB: avoid live vaccines. If never had chickenpox, avoid exposure.

Interactions
Apply to all systemic Rx. fx can be ↓d by rifampicin, carbamazepine,
phenytoin and phenobarbital. fx can be ↑d by erythromycin,
ketoconazole, itraconazole and ciclosporin (whose own fx are ↑d by
methylprednisolone). ↑risk of ↓K⁺ with amphotericin and digoxin.

Withdrawal effects
Acute adrenal insufficiency (= Addisonian crisis; ☠can be fatal☠
see p. 190), ↓BP, fever, myalgia, arthralgia, rhinitis, conjunctivitis,
painful itchy nodules, ↓Wt. ∴ must withdraw slowly if patient has
had >3 wks Rx (or a shorter course w/in 1 year of stopping
long-term Rx), other causes of adrenal suppression, received high

doses (>40 mg od prednisolone or equivalent), or repeat doses in evening, or repeat course. Also note intercurrent illness, trauma, surgery needs ↑doses and can precipitate relative withdrawal.

Steroid Rx card must be carried by all patients on prolonged Rx.

MINERALOCORTICOIDS e.g. fludrocortisone

Used for Addison's disease and acute adrenocortical deficiency (rarely needed for hypopituitarism). Can also be used for orthostatic/postural hypotension. Main SEs are H_2O/Na^+ retention.

SEDATION/SLEEPING TABLETS

ACUTE SEDATION/RAPID TRANQUILLISATION

For the acutely agitated, disturbed or violent patient (and for temporary sedation before unpleasant procedures).

Important points

- Organic causes are commonest cause outside of Ψ wards: look for and treat sepsis, hypoxia, drug withdrawal (esp alcohol/opiates) and metabolic causes (esp hypoglycaemia).
- A well-lit calm room and reassurance can be all that is required.
- Oral medications should be tried first if possible.
- Obtain as much drug Hx as possible, esp of antipsychotics and benzodiazepines as influences selection of appropriate agent/dose.

There are two main choices: antipsychotics and benzodiazepines:
☺ good for/reasons to choose; ☹ bad for/reasons to not give.

Antipsychotics

- ☺ Taking benzodiazepines, elderly or psychotic features (e.g. Schneiderian 1st-rank symptoms or Hx of schizophrenia).
- ☹ Antipsychotic-naive, alcohol withdrawal, cardiac disease, movement disorders (esp Parkinson's. Extrapyramidal fx are common – treat with procyclidine).

- *Haloperidol* 0.5–5 mg po (or im if necessary). 2.5 mg is sensible starting dose for delirium in elderly. 5 mg is safe for acute psychosis in young patients. Maximum 18 mg im or 30 mg po in 24 h (write up prn).
- If suspect *acute schizophrenia*, NICE guidelines now recommend atypical antipsychotic as 1st-line, e.g. olanzapine 10 mg po (⇒ ↓SEs) – now also available im.

Benzodiazepines

☺ Alcohol withdrawal, anxiety, at night time (are 'hypnotic').

☹ Respiratory disease (esp COPD/asthma), elderly (⇒ falls and rarely paradoxical agitation/aggression).

- *Lorazepam* 0.5–1 mg po/im/iv (maximum 4 mg/24 h). Shorter acting than diazepam ∴ better if hepatic impairment.
- *Diazepam* 2–5 mg po/iv (if iv preferably as Diazemuls) or 10–20 mg pr. ↑doses if tolerance/much previous exposure to benzodiazepines.
- *Midazolam* 1.0–7.5 mg iv: titrate up slowly, according to response. Requires iv access and is used mostly for cooperative patients ahead of unpleasant procedures (less suitable for very agitated patients). Also wears off relatively quickly.

SLEEPING TABLETS

Try to avoid giving:

- regularly (dependency common);
- at all if hepatic encephalopathy or ↓respiratory reserve (esp asthma/COPD; NB: *hypoxia can also* ⇒ *restlessness and agitation!*).

Benzodiazpines/Cyclopyrrolones: most commonly used but are addictive and can ⇒ respiratory depression:

- *Temazepam* 10 mg nocte (if tolerant to benzodiazepines, may need 20 mg).
- *Zopiclone* 7.5 mg nocte (NB: start at 3.75 mg if LF (CI if severe), RF or elderly). Can ↑ to 12.5 mg if necessary.

Sedating antihistamines: are a good alternative: ⇒ ↓respiratory depression/addiction but ↑hangover drowsiness; effectiveness may ↓ after several days of Rx ∴ good for inpatients as short-term Rx.

- *Promethazine* 25 mg nocte (can ↑dose to 50 mg)

BENZODIAZEPINES

Varying pharmacokinetics are utilised. If shorter-acting, ⇒ ↓hangover fx (drowsiness) but ⇒ ↑withdrawal fx when stopped.

$t_{1/2}$ (h)	Drug	Use
2	Midazolam	Temporary sedation for painful or stressful procedures; easy iv titration
8	Lorazepam	Emergency epilepsy Rx, acute Ψ sedation; quick-acting, can be given im/iv
10	Temazepam	Sleeping tablet; ↓hangover drowsiness
30	Diazepam	Anxiety (including alcohol withdrawal), emergency epilepsy Rx (short-term)
40	Chlordiazepoxide	Alcohol withdrawal regimes
50	Clonazepam	Movement disorders (especially drug-/neuroleptic-induced), epilepsy and Ψ disorders

ADVERSE EFFECTS

> ☠*Respiratory depression*☠
> Especially in elderly and if naive to benzodiazepines. Put on close nursing observations and monitor O_2 sats if concerned. If using very high doses, get iv access and have flumazenil at hand.

- *Dependence/tolerance:* common ∴ prescribe long-term benzodiazepines *only if absolutely necessary* and withdraw ASAP. In order to withdraw safely, if not already on one, swap to long-acting drug (e.g. diazepam) and take 1/8 off the dose every 2 weeks. Try β-blockers to reduce anxiety (avoid antipsychotics).
- *Withdrawal symptoms:* rebound insomnia, tremor, anxiety, confusion, anorexia, toxic psychosis, convulsions, sweating.

SIDE-EFFECT PROFILES

Knowledge of these, together with a drug's mechanism(s), will simplify learning and allow anticipation of drug SEs.

CHOLINOCEPTORS

ACh stimulates nicotinic and muscarinic receptors. Anticholinesterases $\Rightarrow \uparrow$ ACh and $\therefore$ stimulate both receptor types and have 'cholinergic fx'. Drugs that $\downarrow$ cholinoceptor action do so mostly via muscarinic receptors (antinicotinics used only in anaesthesia) and are $\therefore$ more accurately called 'antimuscarinics' rather than 'anticholinergics'.

Cholinergic fx	Antimuscarinic fx
Generally $\uparrow$ secretions	*Generally $\downarrow$ secretions*
Diarrhoea	**C**onstipation
Urination	**U**rinary retention
Miosis (constriction)	**M**ydriasis/$\downarrow$ accommodation*
Bronchospasm/Bradycardia**	**B**ronchodilation/Tachycardia
Excitation of CNS (and muscle)	**D**rowsiness, **D**ry eyes, **D**ry skin
Lacrimation $\uparrow$	
Saliva/Sweat $\uparrow$	
Commonly caused by:	
Anticholinesterases:	Atropine/ipratropium (Atrovent)
MG Rx, e.g. pyridostigmine	Antihistamines (inc cyclizine)
Dementia Rx, e.g. rivastigmine, donepezil	Antidepressants (esp TCAs)
	Antipsychotics (esp 'typicals')
	Hyoscine, Ia antiarrhythmics

*$\Rightarrow$ blurred vision and $\uparrow$ IOP. **Together with vasodilation $\Rightarrow \downarrow$ BP.

ADRENOCEPTORS

α generally excites sympathetic system (except):*

$\alpha_1 \Rightarrow$ GI smooth-muscle relaxation*, otherwise contracts smooth muscle: vasoconstriction, GI/bladder sphincter constriction (uterus, seminal tract, iris (radial muscle)). Also ↑salivary secretion, ↓glycogenolysis (in liver).

$\alpha_2 \Rightarrow$ inhibition of neurotransmitters (esp NA and ACh for feedback control), Pt aggregation, contraction of vascular smooth muscle, inhibition of insulin release. Also prominent adrenoceptor of CNS (inhibits sympathetic outflow).

β generally inhibits sympathetic system (except*):

$\beta_1 \Rightarrow$ ↑HR*, ↑contractility* (and ↑s salivary amylase secretion).

$\beta_2 \Rightarrow$ Vasodilation, bronchodilation, muscle tremor, glycogenolysis (in hepatic and skeletal muscle). Also ↑s renin secretion, relaxes ciliary muscle and visceral smooth muscles (GI sphincter, bladder detrusor, uterus if not pregnant).

$\beta_3 \rightarrow$ lipolysis, thermogenesis (of little pharmacological relevance).

CEREBELLAR EFFECTS

Esp antiepileptics (e.g. phenytoin) and alcohol.

- **D**ysdiadokokinesis, dysmetria (= past-pointing) and rebound.
- **A**taxia of gait (wide-based, irregular step length) ± trunk.
- **N**ystagmus: towards side of lesion; mostly coarse and horizontal.
- **I**ntention tremor (also titubation = nodding-head tremor).
- **S**peech: scanning dysarthria – slow, slurred or jerky.
- **H**ypotonia (less commonly hyporeflexia or pendular reflexes).

EXTRAPYRAMIDAL EFFECTS

Abnormalities of movement control arising from dysfunction of basal ganglia.

- *Parkinsonism:* rigidity and bradykinesia ± tremor.
- *Dyskinesias* (= abnormal involuntary movements): commonly:
  - *Dystonia* (= abnormal posture): dynamic (e.g. oculogyric crisis) and static (e.g. torticollis).
  - *Tardive (delayed onset) dyskinesia:* esp orofacial movements.
  - *Others:* tremor, chorea, athetosis, hemiballismus, myoclonus, tics.
- *Akathisia* (= restlessness): esp after large antipsychotic doses.

All are commonly caused by antipsychotics (esp older 'typical' drugs) and are a rare complication of antiemetics (e.g. metoclopramide, prochlorperazine – esp in young women). Dyskinesias and dystonias are common with antiparkinsonian drugs (esp peaks of L-dopa doses).

Most respond to stopping (or ↓dose of) the drug – if not possible, doesn't work or immediate Rx needed add antimuscarinic drug (e.g. procyclidine) but doesn't work for akithisia (try β-blocker) and can worsen tardive dyskinesia: seek neurology ± psychiatry opinion if in doubt.

CYTOCHROME P450

Inhibitors	Inducers
Heart/liver failure	Cigarettes
Omeprazole	**P**henytoin
Fluoxetine/**F**luconazole	**C**arbamazepine
Disulfiram	**B**arbiturates (e.g. phenobarbital)
Erythromycin	**R**ifampicin
Valproate	**A**lcohol (chronic abuse*)
Isoniazid	**S**ulphonylureas/**S**t John's wort
Cimetidine/**C**iprofloxacin	
EtOH (acute abuse – note *chronic* abuse can induce!*)	
Sulphonamides	

Substrates of P450 that often result in significant interactions:

- Inhibitors and inducers affect warfarin, phenytoin and theophyllines.
- Inhibitors affect ciclosporin.
- Inducers affect OCP and carbamazepine.

NB: many isoenzymes exist, and the P450 system is very complex, e.g. drugs such as carbamazepine can autoinduce – look for **P450** warning symbols throughout this book.

Medical emergencies

Acute MI (AMI) and acute coronary syndrome (ACS)	178
Acute LVF	181
Accelerated hypertension	181
Anaphylaxis	182
Acute asthma	182
COPD exacerbation	183
Pulmonary embolism	184
Epilepsy	185
DKA	186
HONK	187
↓Glucose	188
Thyrotoxic crisis	188
Myxoedema coma	189
Addisonian crisis	190
Electrolyte disturbances	190
Overdoses	192
Coma	197
Common laboratory reference values	197

!! This section is intended only as a reminder/checklist. It is not a complete guide to Mx, which can be found in other sources and online (e.g. www.eboncall.org). Local Rx preferences and individuality of patients/diseases mean that it is impossible to outline the perfect Rx for every occasion: *always seek senior help if unsure!* ☠ In all emergencies, first follow *ABC + Disability (GCS) + Exposure*. Obtain as much Hx and perform as much examination as is possible. Take time to think and assess: it is more far more common that things go wrong due to a lack of thinking than lack of action. ☠

ACUTE MI (AMI) AND ACUTE CORONARY SYNDROME (ACS)

Clues: angina, N&V, sweating, LVF (see p. 181), ↓BP, Hx of IHD. Remember atypical pain and silent infarcts in DM, elderly and if ↓GCS.

FOR ALL AMI AND ACS

- O_2: maximal flow through re-breather mask (care if COPD).
- *Aspirin:* 300 mg po stat (chew/dispersible form) unless CI. If in A&E, check has not given already by paramedics or GP.
- *Diamorphine:* 2.5–5 mg iv + antiemetic (e.g. metoclopramide 10 mg iv). Repeat diamorphine iv according to response.
- *GTN:* 2 sprays or tablets sl prn. If pain continues or LVF develops, set up ivi, titrating to BP and pain. NB: can ⇒ ↓BP; stop if systolic <100 mmHg (if initial BP high, then hypotensive fx can be useful).

DATE/ TIME	INFUSION FLUID	VOL-UME	ADDITIVES IF ANY DRUG AND DOSE	RATE OF ADMIN	DURA-TION	DR'S SIGNATURE	TIME START-ED	TIME COM-PLETED	SET UP BY SIG-NATURE	BATCH No.
25/12	N. Saline	50 ml	50 mg GTN	0–10 ml/hr*		TN				
	"TITRATE TO PAIN: Stop if systolic BP < 100 mmHg									

Figure 9 Drug chart, showing how to write up GTN ivi.

Consider:

- *β-blocker:* unless CI (see propranolol p. 102), esp beware
  ☠ asthma, acute LVF ☠, ↓BP (systolic <100 mmHg), ↓HR
  (<60/min), 2nd-/3rd-degree HB; get senior help if in doubt.
  - *Can be given iv or po:* it is often recommended to give iv for
    AMI and po for ACS. Consult local protocol or get senior
    advice if unsure.
  - *iv:* e.g. metoprolol 5 mg iv over 5 min. Repeat 5 min later if
    HR still >70 and again 5 min later if HR still >70. Then start
    metoprolol po.
  - *po:* e.g. metoprolol 12.5–50 mg tds. If cardiodynamically stable
    24 h later, change to atenolol 50 mg od and then give bd if
    tolerated.
  - In acute settings, metoprolol is preferred to atenolol as short
    $t_{1/2}$ means it will wear off quicker if LVF develops.
  - If already on β-blocker ensure dose adequate to control HR.
    If β-blocker CI and ↑HR get senior/cardiology advice.
- *Insulin:* for all type I DM and type II DM or non-diabetics with
  CBG >11 on admission. Give conventional sliding scale or GIK
  ivi (e.g. DIGAMI) if local protocol exists; contact CCU for advice.

IF AMI

- *Thrombolysis:* see pp. 161–3 for indications, CIs and choice of
  agent. NB: if appropriate, initiate ASAP during the above steps.
- *Heparin:* iv heparin is always given with recombinant
  thrombolytics for 24–48 h (see p. 163), but not with streptokinase.
  Heparin/LMWH is not usually required after thrombolysis,
  but if ongoing chest pain or ECG Δs get senior advice. If not
  thrombolysed, give LMWH (e.g. enoxaparin 1 mg/kg bd sc or
  dalteparin 120 units/kg bd sc) or iv heparin if PCI a possibility.
- Consider (consult local protocol/cardiology on-call if unsure):
  - *Angioplasty (PCI):* either 'primary' (thrombolysis contra-
    indicated or PCI considered preferable) or 'rescue' (thrombolysis
    does not ↓pain or settle ECG Δs); consult cardiology on call
    for advice.

- *Glycoprotein IIb/IIIa inhibitor:* esp if not thrombolysed (contraindicated or presentation too late) or PCI planned w/in 72 h and still unstable. Use with caution (esp <48 h post-thrombolysis).
- *iv fluids:* if RV infarct. Clues: inferior ECG Δs, ↓BP, ↑JVP, no pulmonary oedema. If suspected, do right-sided ECG and look for ↑ST in V4. Avoid vasodilating drugs (nitrates, opiates, diuretics, ACE-i).

IF ACS (NSTEMI OR UNSTABLE ANGINA)

- *Heparin:* LMWH, e.g. enoxaparin 1 mg/kg bd sc or dalteparin 120 units/kg bd sc (or iv heparin if PCI a possibility).
- Consider (consult local protocol/cardiology on-call if unsure):
  - *Glycoprotein IIb/IIIa inhibitor:* esp if awaiting PCI or if high risk (defined by ESC as*: persistent or recurrent ischaemia, ST depression, DM, ↑troponin, haemodynamic or arrhythmic instability). Local preference of agent varies. NB: expensive, ↑risk of bleeding.
  - *Clopidogrel:* 300 mg po loading dose, then 75 mg od. ESC guidelines recommend for all high-risk patients*, esp if PCI planned.

SECONDARY PREVENTION

For all AMI and ACS unless CI or already started:

- *Next day:* aspirin 75 mg od and statin (e.g. atorvastatin 40 mg od – recent evidence shows ↑ benefit from 80 mg).
- *When stable:* β-blocker (if not already started, e.g. atenolol 50 mg od once any LVF clears; see above for CI) and ACE-i (e.g. ramipril 2.5 mg bd po started 3–10 days after MI, then 5 mg bd after 2 days if tolerated).
- *ASAP:* diet/lifestyle Δs (↓Wt, diet Δs, ↑exercise, ↓smoking, etc.).

ACUTE LVF

Clues: SOB, S_3 or S_4, pulmonary oedema (basal crepts), Hx of IHD, ↑JVP (if also RVF i.e. CCF).

- 60–100% O_2 and sit patient upright.
- Furosemide 60 mg iv; consider ivi later.
- Diamorphine 2.5–5.0 mg iv + metoclopramide 10 mg iv.
- GTN ivi: see Acute MI, p. 178.

If patient does not respond/worsens, consider (and get senior help):

- *Non-invasive ventilation* (NIV) as continuous positive airways pressure (CPAP). If no machine on ward, find one ASAP!
- *Inotropes:* if ↓BP, e.g. dobutamine via central line; if patient is this sick, will also be needed for CVP measurement. Get senior help if needed.
- *?Underlying cause:* MI, arrhythmias (esp AF), severe HTN, ↓↓Hb, ARF, anaphylaxis, sepsis, ARDS, poisons/OD (e.g. aspirin).
- *ACE-i:* once stable and if no CI, e.g. enalapril 2.5–5 mg od.

ACCELERATED HYPERTENSION

Dx if systolic >220 mmHg, diastolic >120 mmHg, or end-organ damage (see p. 137).
☠Do not drop BP too quickly as can ⇒ blindness, CVA and ARF.☠

- *Nifedipine retard* 10–20 mg po: do not give as quick-acting capsules.
- If nifedipine CI, consider β-blocker* (e.g. atenolol 50 mg po) or diuretic (e.g. bendroflumethiazide 2.5 mg po).
- Consider adding atenolol* 50 mg po if IHD or ↑HR.

  *Beware of phaeochromocytoma: if suspected (BP very variable, headaches, sweats, palpitations), give α-blocker (e.g. phenoxy-benzamine, doxazosin) ideally for 2 days before giving β-blocker.

Get senior advice if concerned. Give iv preparations only if patient unconscious and monitored closely (i.e. on ITU). Choose from: GTN/ISDN (esp if LVF), nitroprusside (can $\Rightarrow$ cyanide poisoning), labetalol (can cause severe $\downarrow$BP) or phentolamine.

ANAPHYLAXIS

Clues: bronchoconstriction (SOB, wheeze, stridor), peripheral vasodilation, $\downarrow$BP, arrhythmias, swelling/angioedema, rash, D&V, Hx of asthma, obvious cause (esp recent drugs/iv contrasts).

- 60–100% O_2 (+ secure airway); stop any ivi if possible cause.
- Adrenaline (epinephrine) 0.5 mg *im** (= 0.5 ml of 1:1000 solution). Repeat after 5 min if no clinical improvement.
- Chlorphenamine 10–20 mg iv over 1 min (or im).
- Hydrocortisone 200 mg iv (or im).

Consider:

- iv fluids if $\downarrow$BP persists.
- Salbutamol 5 mg neb if bronchoconstriction persists.
- Intubation if airway compromised (bleep anaesthetist on-call).

> ☠iv* adrenaline (epinephrine) can $\Rightarrow$ arrhythmias ∴ im is preferred route for anaphylaxis unless cardiac arrest seems imminent or concerns over im absorption, in which case give 0.5 mg *iv* (= 5 ml of 1:10 000 (100 μg/ml)) at 1 ml/min until response. *Note iv solution is different strength to im preparations.* ☠

ACUTE ASTHMA

Clues: SOB, wheeze, PEF <50% of best**, RR >25/min, HR >110/min, cannot complete sentences in 1 breath.

- Attach sats monitor.
- 40–60% O_2 through high-flow mask, e.g. Hudson mask.
- Salbutamol 5 mg neb in O_2: repeat up to every 15 min if life threatening.

- Ipratropium 0.5 mg neb in O_2: repeat up to every 4 h if life threatening or fails to respond to salbutamol.
- Prednisolone 40 mg po od for at least 5 days. Hydrocortisone 100 mg qds iv can be given if unable to swallow or retain tablets.

Both prednisolone and hydrocortisone can be given if very ill.

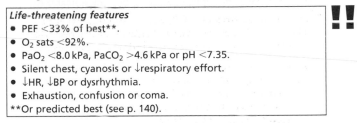

Life-threatening features
- PEF <33% of best**.
- O_2 sats <92%.
- PaO_2 <8.0 kPa, $PaCO_2$ >4.6 kPa or pH <7.35.
- Silent chest, cyanosis or ↓respiratory effort.
- ↓HR, ↓BP or dysrhythmia.
- Exhaustion, confusion or coma.
- **Or predicted best (see p. 140).

If life-threatening features (NB: patient may not always *appear* distressed); get senior help and consider the following:

- *$MgSO_4$ ivi*: 8 mmol over 20 min (= 2 g = 4 ml of 50% solution).
- *Aminophylline iv*: attach cardiac monitor and give loading dose* of 5 mg/kg iv over 20 min then ivi at 0.5–0.7 mg/kg/h.
  If already taking maintenance po aminophylline/ theophylline, omit loading dose* and check levels ASAP to guide dosing.
- *iv salbutamol*: 5 µg/min initially (then up to 20 µg/min according to response): back-to-back or continuous nebs now often preferred.
- Call anaesthetist for consideration of ITU care or intubation. Initiate this during the above steps if deteriorating.

COPD EXACERBATION

Clues: SOB, wheeze, RR >25/min, HR >110.

- *Attach sats monitor* and do baseline ABGs.
- *28% O_2 via Venturi mask*; should be *prescribed on drug chart*. ↑dose cautiously if hypoxia continues, but repeat ABGs to ensure CO_2 not ↑ing and (more importantly) pH not ↓ing.

- *Ipratropium 0.5 mg neb* in O_2: repeat up to every 4 h if very ill.
- *Salbutamol 5 mg neb* in O_2: repeat up to every 15 min if very ill (seldom necessary >hourly).
- *Prednisolone 30 mg po* then od for ≤2 wks (some give 1st dose as hydrocortisone 200 mg iv; rarely used now unless unable to swallow).
- *Antibiotics* (see p. 132) if 2 out of 3 of Hx of ↑ing SOB, ↑ing volume or ↑ing purulence of sputum.

If no improvement, consider:

- *Aminophylline ivi:* see management of asthma (p. 183) for details.
- Assisted ventilation: CPAP if just ↓PaO_2 or NIV (BIPAP) if also ↑$PaCO_2$; consider doxapram if NIV not available.
- Intubation: discuss with ITU/anaesthetist.

PULMONARY EMBOLISM

Clues: unlikely unless RR >20 and PaO_2 <10.7 kPa (or ↓O_2 sats).

- *60–100% O_2* if hypoxic. Care if COPD.
- *Analgesia:* if xs pain or distress, try paracetamol/ibuprofen first; consider opiates if severe or no response (☠ can ⇒ respiratory depression ☠).
- *Anticoagulation:* LMWH, e.g. dalteparin or enoxaparin.
  Once PE confirmed, load with warfarin (see pp. 155–7). Consider iv heparin if surgery being contemplated, or rapid reversal may be required*.

If massive PE, worsening hypoxia or cardiovascular instability (↓BP, RV strain/failure), seek senior help and consider:

- *Fluids ± inotropes:* if systolic BP <90 mmHg.
- *Thrombolysis (e.g. alteplase):* if ↓BP ± collapse.
- *Embolectomy*:* seek urgent cardiothoracic opinion.

EPILEPSY

Status epilepticus = seizures for >30 min or >1 episode w/o full recovery in between. NB: non-convulsive/absence seizures are missed easily. Keep in mind non-epileptic (= pseudo) seizures, esp if atypical fits or past Ψ Hx.

- *Protect airway:* get senior help early if concerned.
- *Attach O_2 sats monitor* and *place in recovery position.*
- 60–100% O_2 (beware COPD).
- *Exclude or treat reversible metabolic causes:* esp ↓O_2, glucose, ↓thiamine (esp if alcoholic), ↓pyridoxine.
- *Diazepam 10 mg iv* over 2 min, preferable as Diazemuls (↓s thrombophlebitis), repeating if necessary at 5 mg/min to maximum of 20 mg. If no iv access, give 30 mg pr. ☠Beware respiratory depression.☠
- *Check BP:* maintain or ↑mean arterial blood pressure to provide appropriate cerebral perfusion pressure: get senior help if concerned.

If no response get senior help and give:

- *Lorazepam ivi:* 0.1 mg/kg at 2 mg/min (can use lower rate of infusion). If not available on ward, give diazepam ivi: 100 mg in 500 ml 5% glucose at 40 ml/h.

If no response after 10 min, call for anaesthetist and give:

- *Phenytoin iv:* see p. 99 for dose. Monitor BP and HR (both can drop) and ECG (esp QTc, as arrhythmias not uncommon). Phenobarbital 10–15 mg/kg iv at 100 mg/min is an alternative.

If the above measures do not terminate seizures, refractory status epilepticus is present. Requires general anaesthesia with propofol or thiopental in a specialised unit.

DKA

Clues: ketotic breath, Kussmaul's (deep/rapid) breathing, dehydration, confusion/↓GCS.

- *Initial measures:* O_2 if hypoxic, insert NGT if coma, weigh patient (if possible). Consider central line (esp if ↓↓pH or Hx of HF), but urinary catheter often sufficient (insert if no urine after 2–3 h).
- *iv fluids:* initially 0.9% saline according to individual patient needs (guided by urine output ± CVP). The following is a guide:
  - *If severe dehydration,* i.e. shock, oliguria or ARF (in this context = urea >21 mmol/l or creatinine >350 mmol/l), give 1st litre over 30 min, 2nd litre over 1 h and 3rd litre over 2 h. Consider colloid if ↓↓BP or no improvement in hydration.
  - *Otherwise* give more slowly, e.g. 2 l over 4 h, then 1 l over 4 h.
  - Add KCl once K^+ <5.5 mmol/l, as can ↓rapidly dt insulin (but do not give KCl in 1st litre unless K^+ <3.5 mmol/l). Roughly 20–30 mmol needed per litre during rehydration: adjust to individual response with regular checks (easiest and quickest done with ABG machines: most give K^+ levels, and ABGs also needed regularly for pH monitoring; can also use venous samples as long as put in ABG or other heparinised syringe).
- *Insulin:* as soluble insulin ivi (e.g. Actrapid). A sensible start is 6 units/h, ↑ing to 12 units/h if no ↓BG w/in 2 h. Higher doses can ⇒ too rapid a fall in BG and K^+ (aim for ↓BG of 3–6 mmol/h). If no ivi facilities available, give 10 units iv stat (↓dose if BG <20). Once BG <12, change iv fluids to 5% glucose and start insulin sliding scale (see p. 153), adjusting to response but ideally maintaining min rate of 4 units/h with sufficient glucose ivi (if insulin continued, speed of ketone clearance ↑s; if BG <5, do not stop insulin but ↑rate of glucose ivi or switch to 10% solution). Continue until ketones cleared (check urine ± blood), pH normal and eating/drinking; then switch to sc regime (see p. 153 for advice).
- *Heparin:* if comatose or hyperosmolar (>350 mosmol/l), give LMWH (or unfractionated heparin 5000 units sc bd/tds). Continue until mobile.

Consider:

- *Antibiotics:* search for and treat infection. NB: rely on CRP more than WCC (WCC can be artificially ↑d) and temperature can be normal even in severe infections ∴ dipstick urine and send urine, blood and any other relevant cultures (consider CXR). If suspect infection and no clear cause, start blind Rx, e.g. cefotaxime 1 g bd iv (or other 3rd-generation cephalosporin).
- *Bicarbonate:* if severe acidosis (e.g. pH <7); very rarely needed and potentially dangerous. Get senior help if concerned.
- *HDU/ITU:* for one-to-one nursing ± ventilation if required.

Watch for complications: *electrolyte Δs* (esp ↓Na$^+$, ↓K$^+$, ↓Mg^{++}, ↓PO$_4$), TE (esp DVT/PE), *cerebral oedema* (↓GCS, papilloedema, false-localising cranial nerve palsies), *infections* (esp aspiration pneumonia).

HONK

Clues: as for DKA, but no ketones, normal pH, ↑glucose, ↑dehydration and ↑confusion. Generally ↑age of patient and ↑length of Hx of decline (NB: may be 1st presentation and no past Hx). Can also be precipitated by steroids and thiazides.

- *Initial measures:* as DKA, see p. 186.
- *iv fluids:* as DKA, but can correct dehydration more slowly (will have occurred more slowly and also ↓s risk of electrolyte abnormalities). A rough guide is 1 l of 0.9% saline over 1 h, then 2 l over 4 h ×2, then 1 l over 4 h. Less KCl will be needed, as less insulin will be used. NB: can remain in circulatory collapse despite clinically adequate fluid replacement; if so, give 500 ml colloid and monitor CVP. Consider 0.45% saline if Na$^+$ >155 mmol/l; get senior (ideally specialist) help first.
- *Insulin:* start at lower dose than DKA (e.g. 2 units/h ivi). Again aim to ↓BG by 3–6 mmol/h and continue ivi for ⩾24 h (adding glucose if necessary to keep BG normal) before switching to sc regime.

- *Heparin:* iv or LMWH (see pp. 159–61). Always give, as ↑↑osmolality ⇒ ↑risk of TE (and consider TEDS).

Consider:

- *Antibiotics:* search for and treat infection, as above.

Watch for complications, esp TE (CVA, IHD) and ARF.

↓GLUCOSE

Treat if <2.5 mmol/l or symptoms: ↑sympathetic drive (↑HR, sweating, aggression/behavioural Δs), seizures or confusion/↓GCS.

- *Glucose orally:* esp sugary drinks or mouth gel (e.g. Hypostop). Miss this step if severe, but can be useful if delays in iv access.
- *Glucose 20–50 ml of 50%* iv stat via large Venflon. Always flush liberally with saline as 50% glucose is very viscous and will act slowly otherwise. Repeat if necessary. A brisk 5–20% glucose ivi can be used if only mild symptoms or until 50% glucose found, but beware of fluid overload if HF.
- *Glucagon 1 mg* im/iv stat: if very low glucose or no iv access.

  NB: think of and correct any causes, esp xs DM Rx, alcohol withdrawal, liver failure, aspirin OD (rarely Addison's disease, ↓T4).

THYROTOXIC CRISIS

Clues: ↑HR/AF, fever, abdominal pain, D&V, tremor, agitation, confusion, coma. Look for goitre, Grave's eye disease.

- *O₂:* if hypoxic.
- *0.9% saline ivi:* slowly as per individual needs (care if HF).
- *Propranolol 40 mg tds po:* aim for HR <100 and titrate up dose if necessary (if β-blocker CI, give diltiazem 60–120 mg qds po). If ↑↑HR, give propranolol iv 1 mg over 1 min, repeating if necessary every 2 min to max total of 10 mg.

- *Digoxin and LMWH* (if AF): DC shock rarely works until euthyroid ∴ load with 500 µg iv over 30 min then 250 µg iv over 30 min every 2 h until HR <100 (up to max total of 1.5 mg).
- *Carbimazole:* 15–30 mg qds po (↓ later under specialist advice).
- *Lugol's solution (iodine):* 0.1–0.3 ml tds po (normally for 1 wk). Start 4 h after carbimazole.
- *Hydrocortisone:* 100 mg qds iv (or dexamethasone 4 mg qds po).

Consider:

- *Treat any heart failure* (common if fast AF), e.g. furosemide.
- *Antibiotics:* if evidence/suspicion of infection, e.g. 3rd-generation cephalosporin iv, such as cefotaxime 1 g bd iv.
- *Cooling measures:* paracetamol, sponging.

If vomiting, insert NGT to avoid aspiration and for drug administration.

MYXOEDEMA COMA

Clues: 'facies', goitre, thyroidectomy scar, ↓temperature, ↓HR, ↓reflexes, ↓glucose, seizures, coma. NB: Ψ features common.

- O_2: if hypoxic.
- *Glucose iv:* if hypoglycaemic (often coexists); see p. 188.
- *0.9% saline ivi:* slowly as per individual needs (care if HF).
- *Liothyronine* (= T_3 = tri-iodothyronine): 5–20 µg ivi bd for ≥2 days then ↑dose gradually with endocrinologist's advice before converting to thyroxine po. Liothyronine can precipitate angina; slow down ivi if occurs.
- *Hydrocortisone:* 100 mg iv tds, esp if suspect hypopituitarism (much more likely if no goitre or past Hx of Rx for ↑T_4).

Consider:

- *Rewarming measures:* e.g. Bair-Hugger, warmed fluids (and O_2).
- *Antibiotics:* infections are common and may have precipitated decline ∴ have low threshold for aggressive Rx (e.g. iv 3rd-generation cephalosporin).
- *Ventilation/ITU:* condition has high mortality.

ADDISONIAN CRISIS

Clues: ↓BP, ↑HR, ↓glucose, ↑K$^+$/↓Na$^+$, Hx of chronic high-dose steroid Rx with missed doses or intercurrent illness*?

- O_2 if cyanosed.
- *Glucose iv:* if hypoglycaemic; see p. 188.
- *Hydrocortisone:* 100 mg iv stat then qds (ensure blood sample for cortisol and ACTH taken first if Dx is not certain).
- *Fluids iv:* colloid ± central line if ↓↓BP.
- *Antibiotics:* look for and treat infection*: dipstick urine, MSU, CXR and blood cultures. If in doubt, start Rx (e.g. iv 3rd-generation cephalosporin such as cefotaxime 1 g bd iv).

ELECTROLYTE DISTURBANCES

↑K$^+$

K$^+$ >6 mmol/l is considered dangerous. *Is haemolysis a possibility?* Ring laboratory and repeat sample if suspicious. Treat causes of ↑K$^+$. If K$^+$ >6.5 mmol/l or ECG Δs (tall tented T waves, QRS >0.12 s (>3 small squares), loss of P waves or sinusoidal pattern) the following is also needed:

- *Attach cardiac monitor* (+ECG if possible): risk of arrhythmias.
- *10 ml of 10% Ca^{++} gluconate* iv over 2 min for cardioprotection, or 10 ml of 10% CaCl iv at ≤ 1 ml/min (often in crash trolleys as Min-I-Jet syringes).
- *10 units insulin* (e.g. Actrapid) + 50 ml 50% glucose ivi over 30 min: stimulates cellular membrane H$^+$/K$^+$ pumps ∴ ↓s plasma K$^+$ levels. Beware of too rapid a drop as this may precipitate arrhythmias: aim for drop of 1–2 mmol/l over 30–60 min.
- Consider *salbutamol 5–20 mg nebs:* utilises K$^+$-lowering fx.

For all patients with ↑K$^+$:

- *Look for and treat causes*, esp ARF and drugs (e.g. iv KCl, oral K$^+$ supplements, ACE-i, K$^+$-sparing diuretics, NSAIDs, ciclosporin).

- Calcium Resonium 15 g tds/qds po if ↑K^+ persists. NB: slow action.

↓K^+

<2.5 mmol/l ⇒ risk of arrhythmias: attach cardiac monitor.

- *1 l normal saline (0.9%) + 40 mmol KCl* over 4 h. If unstable or arrhythmias develop, seek senior help. KCl can be given quicker but non-specialist wards may not allow >10 mmol/h and patient may not tolerate fast peripheral ivi due to pain (consider central line).
- *Oral K^+ replacement* should be commenced (e.g. Sando-K, Slow-K 2 tablets tds, or as much as can be tolerated – unpleasant taste!). Beware of overshooting later, esp if cause removed.

NB: po replacement is often sufficient if K^+ >2.5 mmol/l and no clinical features/ECG Δs (small T waves or large U waves).

↑Ca^{++}

>2.65 mmol/l is abnormal. Symptoms usually start once >2.9 mmol/l. *Clues:* bones (pain, esp consider metastases), stones (renal colic ⊥ ARF), groans (abdominal pains, constipation ± vomiting; polyuria and thirst common) and psychic moans (including confusion).

If >3.0 mmol/l or severe symptoms (as above) give:

- *0.9% saline ivi:* average requirements 4–6 l over 24 h (↓ if elderly/HF). Monitor fluid balance carefully and correct electrolytes.

If insufficient improvement in Ca^{++} levels or symptoms consider:

- *Bisphosphonate* (e.g. pamidronate) esp if ↑PTH or malignancy.
- *Calcitonin:* if no response to bisphosphonate.
- *Steroids:* if sarcoid, lymphoma, myeloma or vitamin D toxicity.
- *Forced saline diuresis* (high-volume saline + furosemide) if severely ill (e.g. coma, arrhythmias). Consider dialysis if ARF. Get senior help.

OVERDOSES

Unless you are familiar with the up-to-date Mx of the specific overdose in question, the following sources should always be consulted:

- *Toxbase website (www.spib.axl.co.uk):* authoritative and updated regularly. Should be used in the 1st instance to check clinical features and Mx of the poison(s) in question. You will need to sign in under your departmental account; if your department is not registered, contact your A&E department to obtain a username and password.
- *National Poisons Information Service (NPIS):* tel. 0870 600 6266 for advice if unsure of Toxbase instructions and for rarer/mixed overdoses.

GENERAL MEASURES

- *GI decontamination:* activated charcoal (and, rarely, gastric lavage) can be given if w/in 1 h* of significant OD ingestion. Both are CI if ↓GCS (unless ET tube in situ). Gastric lavage is also CI if corrosive OD or risk of GI haemorrhage/perforation. Activated charcoal can be repeated with certain drugs but does not work with others (most notably, lithium, iron, organophosphates, ethylene glycol, ethanol, methanol). Consult Toxbase ± NPIS for severe or unusual poisoning, as routine GI decontamination is no longer recommended.
- Check paracetamol and aspirin levels in all patients who are unable to give an accurate Hx of the exact poisons ingested.

*Unless drug is MR preparation or causes delayed gastric emptying (e.g. salicylates, opiates, TCAs, theophyllines, sympathomimetics). In such cases, GI decontamination can be given later; exactly how much longer is a controversial issue, so contact NPIS if you are concerned about a potentially serious ingestion. See Toxbase for dosage guide for activated charcoal.

PARACETAMOL

Significant OD = ingestion of 150 mg/kg or 12 g (whichever is smaller). If risk factors (see below), 75 mg/kg should be used instead.

Risk factors in paracetamol OD

- Taking enzyme-inducing drugs, e.g. carbamazepine, phenobarbital, primidone, phenytoin, rifampicin, St John's wort.
- Regularly consumes alcohol in xs of recommended amounts.
- Malnourished and likely to be glutathione-deplete, e.g. anorexia, alcoholism, cystic fibrosis, HIV infection.

Mx depends on time since ingestion:

0–8 h post-ingestion:

- *Activated charcoal*: if w/in 1 h of significant OD.
- *Acetylcysteine*: wait until 4 h post-ingestion before taking urgent sample for paracetamol levels (results are meaningless until this time). If presents at 4–8 h post-ingestion, take sample ASAP. If levels above the treatment line (see below), give the following acetylcysteine regime:
  - *Initially* 150 mg/kg in 200 ml 5% glucose ivi over 15 min.
  - *Then* 50 mg/kg in 500 ml 5% glucose ivi over 4 h.
  - *Then* 100 mg/kg in 115% glucose ivi over 16 h.

Do not delay acetylcysteine beyond 8 h post-ingestion if waiting for paracetamol levels result and significant OD (beyond 8 h, efficacy ↓s substantially) – ivi can be stopped if levels come back as below treatment line and INR, ALT and creatinine normal.

8–15 h post-ingestion:

- *Acetylcysteine*: give above regime ASAP if significant OD taken. Do not wait for paracetamol level result. Acetylcysteine can be stopped if level later turns out to be below treatment line, timing of the OD is certain, and patient asymptomatic with normal INR/creatinine/ALT.

15–24 h post-ingestion:

- *Acetylcysteine:* give above regime ASAP unless certain that significant OD has not been taken. Do not wait for paracetamol level result. Presenting this late ⇒ severe risk, and treatment lines are unreliable: always finish course of acetylcysteine.

>24 h post-ingestion:

- Acetylcysteine is controversial when presenting this late. Monitor as below and discuss the individual case with NPIS.

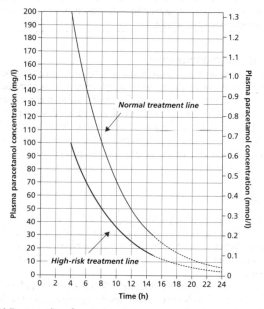

Figure 10 Treatment lines for acetylcysteine treatment of paracetamol overdose. Reproduced courtesy of Alun Hutchings and University of Wales College of Medicine Therapeutics and Toxicology Centre.

NB: use high-risk line if any of the risk factors listed above apply.

> **Important points regarding acetylcysteine**
> - Have lower threshold for initiating Rx if doubts over timing of OD, if ingestion was staggered, if presents 24–36 h post-ingestion, or if evidence of LF/severe toxicity regardless of time since ingestion.
> - If anaphylactoid reactions occurs, stop infusion and give antihistamine (e.g. chlorphenamine 10–20 mg iv over 1 min) and restart acetylcysteine ivi at the next dose down. Ignore past history of adverse reactions, but ensure 1st infusion is at the right dose and speed.

Subsequent management

GCS and urine output should be monitored closely. Patients should be *medically* fit for discharge once acetylcysteine ivi is completed, and INR, ALT, creatinine and HCO_3^- (±pH) subsequently checked to be normal and stable (*psychiatric* clearance for discharge may take longer). If abnormalities detected, consult Toxbase ± NPIS for consideration of further acetylcysteine and specialist referral. On discharge, advise all patients to return to hospital if abdominal pains or vomiting develop.

ASPIRIN

- *Activated charcoal ± gastric lavage:* if w/in 1 h of OD of ≥250 mg/kg. Aspirin delays gastric emptying (esp if enteric-coated tablets), ∴ both can be given >1 h after ingestion and activated charcoal can be repeated later; contact NPIS for advice.
- *Monitor* U&Es, glucose, clotting, ABGs (or venous pH and HCO_3^-) and fluid balance (often need large volumes of iv fluid). Take salicylate levels at 2 h post-ingestion if symptomatic or 4 h post-ingestion if not symptomatic, repeating in both cases 2 h later in case of delayed absorption.

If abnormalities detected, get senior help or contact ITU for specialist advice, and then consider the following:

- *Sodium bicarbonate:* 1.5 l of 1.26% iv over 2 h (or 225 ml of 8.4%). Give only if metabolic acidosis and salicylate levels >500 mg/l. Ensure given through patent cannula (risk of tissue necrosis if extravasation), and must have excluded or corrected ↓K$^+$. Such alkalinisation of urine can itself ↓K$^+$ so iv KCl replacement may be needed; monitor K$^+$ closely (easiest done on ABGs as also need regular monitoring). Consider further 225 ml ivi of 8.4% sodium bicarbonate to keep urine pH at 7.5–8.5.
- *Haemodialysis:* if salicylate levels >700 mg/l (or unresponsive to the above measures), ARF, CCF, non-cardiac pulmonary oedema, severe metabolic acidosis, convulsions or any CNS fx that are not resolved by correction of pH. Have lower threshold if age >70 years.

OPIATES

Clues: pinpoint pupils, ↓respiratory rate, ↓GCS, drug chart and Hx/signs of opiate abuse (e.g. track marks).

- O_2 + maintain airway ± ventilatory support.
- *Naloxone 0.8–2.0 mg iv* (or im) stat: repeat every 2–3 min if needed (maximum total dose 10 mg). NB: short $t_{1/2}$ ∴ consider ivi (rarely needed).

BENZODIAZEPINES

- O_2 + maintain airway ± ventilatory support.
- Consider *flumazenil:* get senior opinion if concerned. See p. 57 for dosage.

> ☠*Flumazenil is not recommended as a diagnostic test and should not be given routinely.* ☠ Risk of inducing fits (esp if epileptic), withdrawal syndrome (if habituated to benzodiazepines) or arrhythmias (esp if coingested TCA or amphetamine-like drug

of abuse). If in any doubt, get senior opinion and never give without normal ECG and excluding patient habituation to benzodiazepines.

COMA

Motor response	Verbal response	Eye opening
6 Obeys commands	5 Orientated	4 Spontaneous
5 Localises pain	4 Confused	3 Responds to speech
4 Withdraws to pain	3 Inappropriate	2 Responds to pain
3 Flexes to pain	2 Incomprehensible	1 None
2 Extends to pain	1 None	
1 No response to pain		

GCS 13–15 = minor injury
GCS 9–12 = moderate injury
GCS <9   = severe injury

NB: drops of ≥2 are often significant.

Causes of ↓GCS = DIM TOPS
- *Drugs:* alcohol, insulin, sedatives, overdoses,
- *Infections:* sepsis, meningitis, encephalitis.
- *Metabolic:* ↑/↓glucose, ↓T_4, RF, LF.
- *Trauma Hx:* especially lucid interval of extradural.
- *O_2 deficiency:* any cause of ↓O_2 (also ↑CO_2).
- *Perfusion:* CVA, including SAH.
- *Seizures:* post-ictal, non-convulsive status.

COMMON LABORATORY REFERENCE VALUES

NB: normal ranges often vary between laboratories. The ranges given here are deliberately narrow to minimise missing abnormal results, but this means that your result may be normal for your laboratory's range, which should always be checked if possible.

Biochemistry

Na$^+$	135–145 mmol/l
K$^+$	3.5–5.0 mmol/l
Urea	2.5–6.5 mmol/l
Creatinine	70–110 μmol/l
Ca^{++}	2.15–2.65 mmol/l
PO$_4$	0.8–1.4 mmol/l
Albumin	35–50 g/l
Protein	60–80 g/l
Mg^{++}	0.75–1.0 mmol/l
Cl$^-$	95–105 mmol/l
Glucose (fasting)	3.5–5.5 mmol/l
LDH	70–250 iu/l
CK	25–195* u/l (↑ in blacks)
Trop I	<0.4 ng/ml (= μg/l)
Trop T	<0.1 ng/ml (= μg/l)
D-dimers	<0.5** mg/l
Bilirubin	3–17 μmol/l
ALP	30–130 iu/l
AST	3–31 iu/l
ALT	3–35 iu/l
GGT	7–50* iu/l
Cholesterol	3.9–5.2 mmol/l
TG	0.5–1.9 mmol/l
Urate	0.2–0.45 mmol/l
Amylase	0–180 u/dl
CRP	0–10 mg/l

Haematology

Hb male	13.5–17.5 g/dl
Hb female	11.5–15.5 g/dl
Pt	150–400 × 10^9/l
WCC	4–11 × 10^9/l

*Sex differences exist: females occupy the lower end of the range.

**D-dimer normal range can vary with different test protocols: check with your lab!

Haematology (Continued)

NØ	$2.0–7.5 \times 10^9$/l (40–75%)
LØ	$1.3–3.5 \times 10^9$/l (20–45%)
EØ	$0.04–0.44 \times 10^9$/l (1–6%)
PCV (= Hct)	0.37–0.54* l/l
MCV	76–96 fl
ESR	<age in years (+ 10 in women)/2
HbA$_{1C}$	2.3–6.5%

Clotting

APTT	35–45 s
APTT ratio	0.8–1.2
INR	0.8–1.2

Haematinics

Iron	11–30 μmol/l
Transferrin	2–4 g/l
TIBC	45–72 μmol/l
Serum folate	1.8–11 μg/l
B$_{12}$	200–760 pg/ml (= ng/l)

Arterial blood gases

PaO$_2$	>10.6 kPa
PaCO$_2$	4.7–6.0 kPa
pH	7.35–7.45
HCO$_3^-$	24–30 mmol/l
Base xs	±2 mmol/l

Thyroid function

Thyroxine (total T$_4$)	70–140 nmol/l
Thyroxine (free T$_4$)	9–22 pmol/l
TSH	0.5–5 mU/l

*Sex differences exist: females occupy the lower end of the range.

INDEX

AAC 133
accelerated hypertension 181–2
acute adrenal insufficiency 190
acute asthma 182–3
acute bronchitis 132
acute coronary syndrome 178–80
acute epiglottitis 132
acute LVF 181
acute myocardial infarction 178–80
acute sedation 171–2
Addisonian crisis 190
adrenoceptors 174–5
AF (ALS algorithm) *see inside back cover*
alcohol withdrawal 147–8
ALS universal algorithm *see outside back cover flap*
analgesia 140–4
anaphylaxis 182
antibiotics 128–37
antibiotic-associated colitis 133
anticoagulants 154–61
anticholinergic side effects (= antimuscarinic side effects) 174
antiemetics 145–6
antimuscarinic side effects 174
aspiration pneumonia 131
aspirin overdose 195–6
asthma
  acute 182–3
  chronic 139–40

atrial fibrillation ALS algorithm *see inside back cover*

benzodiazepines
  general: types/properties 173
  for acute sedation/sleep 172
  overdose of 196
bowel prep(aration)s 17
bradycardia ALS algorithm *see outside front cover flap*
broad complex tachycardia ALS algorithm *see inside front cover*
bronchitis, acute 132
BTS guidelines for asthma Mx 139

cavitating pneumonia 131
cellulitis 136
cerebellar side effects 175
cholinoceptors 174
Clostridium difficile colitis 133
coma 197
community acquired pneumonia 128
conjunctivitis 135
controlled drugs 163
COPD, acute exacerbation 183–4
corticosteroids 169–71
cystic fibrosis, pneumonia 132
cytochrome p450 176

detox regime, for alcohol
147–8
diabetic
control (inc pre-op) *see*
insulin
ketoacidosis 186
diamorphine (sc) pump 142–4
dilating drops (for eyes) 44
DKA 186

electrolyte
acute abnormalities/
emergencies 190–1
fluid Mx 166–9
epiglottitis 132
epilepsy, acute 185
eye infections 135
extrapyramidal side effects
175–6

fluid management 166–9

gastroenteritis 133
GCS (Glasgow Coma Scale)
197
GTN ivi pump 178

Helicobacter pylori eradication
133
heparin
indications/doses/monitoring/
OD 158–61
in thrombolysis 163
HONK 187–8
hospital acquired pneumonia
130

hypercalcaemia
Mx of 191
in palliative care 144
hyperkalaemia 190–1
hyperosmolar non ketotic state
187–8
hypertension
acute/accelerated/malignant
181–2
chronic (choice of agent)
137–9
hyperthyroid storm 188
hypoglycaemia 188
hypokalaemia 191
hypothyroid coma 189

INR 155–6
insulin
types/sliding scales/pre-op
150–4
in DKA 186
iv (intravenous) fluids 166–9

lab reference values, for blood
tests 197–9
left ventricular failure (LVF),
acute Mx 181
low molecular weight heparin
158
LVF (left ventricular failure),
acute Mx 181

malaria 133–4
meningitis 134–5
mineralocorticoids 171
myxoedema (coma) 189

narrow complex tachycardia (NCT) ALS algorithm *see inside front cover flap*
nausea, causes of/Rx of 145–6
neutropenia 137
normal values, of blood tests 197–9

ocular infections 135
opiate overdose 196
osteomyelitis 136
otitis externa/media 132
overdoses 192–7
  aspirin 195–6
  benzodiazepines 196
  general measures 192
  opiates 196
  paracetamol 193–5

pain control 140–4
palliative care 142–4
paracetamol overdose 193–5
PE 184
peak (expiratory) flow (PEF) predictor 140
pneumonias 128–31
  aspiration 131
  cavitating 131
  community acquired 128
  hospital acquired 130
  TB 131
post-op
  analgesia 140–1
  diabetes/insulin/sliding scales 154

potassium
  in iv fluids 167–8
  hyperkalaemia 190–1
  hypokalaemia 191
  tablets 100
pre-op
  diabetes/insulin/sliding scales 154
pulmonary embolism (PE) 184
PUO (pyrexia of unknown origin) 136
pyelonephritis 132
pyrexia of unknown origin 136

rapid tranquillisation 171–3

sedation (acute/sleeping tablets) 171–3
septic arthritis 136
side effect profiles 174–6
sinusitis 132
sleeping tablets 172–3
sliding scales (of insulin) 150–3
status asthmaticus 182–3
status epilepticus 185
steroids 169–71
strep throat 132
streptokinase 161–3
subcutaneous pumps (in palliative care) 142–4
surgery
  analgesia 140–1
  diabetes/insulin/sliding scales 154

TB 131
thrombolysis 161–3
thyrotoxic crisis/storm
      188–9
triple therapy (for *H. pylori*
      eradication) 133
tuberculosis 131

urinary tract infection (UTI) 132
unstable angina (*see* ACS)
      178–80

warfarin: indications/doses/
      monitoring/OD 154–8
Wernicke's encephalopathy 147

Gaviscon: 10-20 ml
    ''   Advance: 5-10 ml

ERCP PRophylaxis: 1g Amoxycillin
once pre-ercp.

                 20mg Gentamicin

Surgery: Cefuroxime I.V. 750 mg TDS
                   PO 500mg ~~TDS~~ BD
       metronidazole I.V. 500 mg TDS
                   PO 400 mg TDS

       CIPROflexacin IV/PO 500mg BD

Buscopan 10-20mg IV/PO/
                 TDS.

Milpar 5-20 mls PRN
Levonelle 1500 mg OD (Morning after Pill)
Lorazepam 1-2 mg max 4 mg
Haloperidol 2-10 mg PO max 30 mg
            2-5 mg IM max 18 mg